FAMILY PLANNING
FOR
MARRIAGE

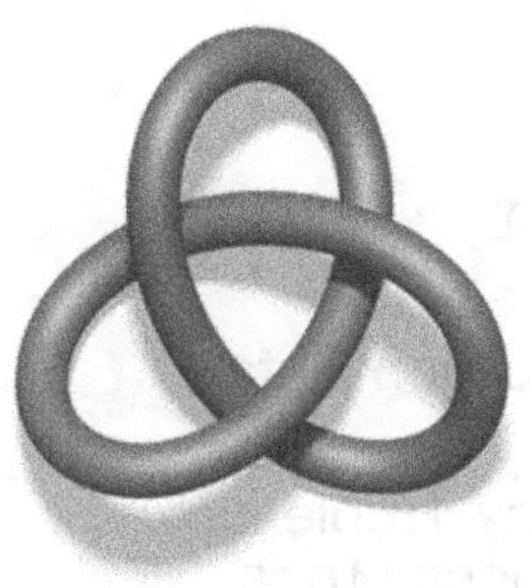

TREBLE-UP
USE THREE FORMS OF BIRTH CONTROL

Treble-Up

ISBN: 978-1-64718-679-1

Published by BookLocker.com, Inc., St. Petersburg, Florida.

Printed on acid-free paper.

BookLocker.com, Inc.
2020

First Edition, 2017, Second Edition 2020

Library of Congress Cataloging in Publication Data
Treble-Up
FAMILY PLANNING FOR MARRIAGE by Treble-Up
Library of Congress Control Number: 2020911015

DISCLAIMER

This book details the author's research and personal opinions about sexual education, contraceptive use and disease prevention. The author is not a health care provider.

The author and publisher are providing this book and its contents on an "as is" basis and make no representations or warranties of any kind with respect to this book or its contents. The author and publisher disclaim all such representations and warranties, including, for example, warranties of merchantability and health care for a particular purpose. In addition, the author and publisher do not represent or warrant that the information accessible via this book is accurate, complete or current.

The statements made about products and services have not been evaluated by the U.S. Food and Drug Administration. They are not intended to diagnose, treat, cure, or prevent any condition or disease. Please consult with your own physician or health care specialist regarding the suggestions and recommendations made in this book.

Except as specifically stated in this book, neither the author nor publisher, nor any authors, contributors, or other representatives will be liable for damages arising out of or in connection with the use of this book. This is a comprehensive limitation of liability that applies to all damages of any kind, including (without limitation) compensatory; direct, indirect or consequential damages; loss of data, income or profit; loss of or damage to property; and claims of third parties.

You understand that this book is not intended as a substitute for consultation with a licensed health care practitioner, such as your physician. Before you begin any health care program, or change your lifestyle in any way, you will consult your physician or other licensed health care practitioner to ensure that you are in good health and that the examples contained in this book will not harm you.

This book provides content related to topics of physical and/or mental health issues. As such, use of this book implies your acceptance of this disclaimer.

Table of Contents

Introduction: Accidental Pregnancy and Why It Matters

The United States has the highest rate of teen pregnancy in the developed world,[1] and Texas is fifth highest in the 50 states,[2] with the highest rate of repeat teen pregnancies![3] That's not surprising, given that 25% of Texas school districts **don't** teach sex education and almost 60% teach abstinence-only.[4]

The figure below shows the 2012 birth rates in teens by state.[5] As you can see, Texas sits right in the middle of a hotbed of teen pregnancy and births, along with New Mexico, Mississippi, Arkansas, Louisiana, Oklahoma, Kentucky and West Virginia.

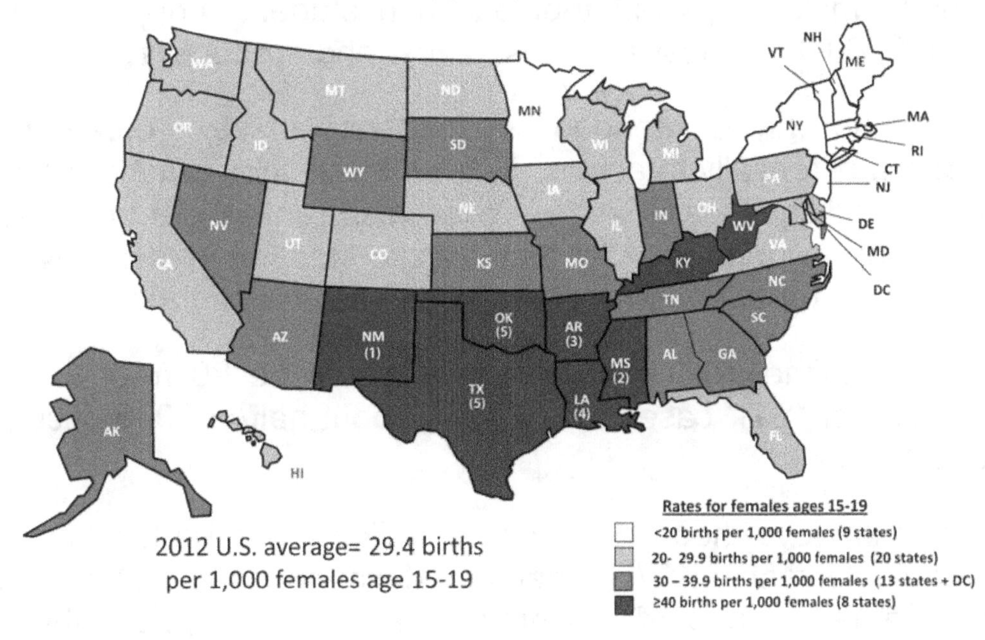

2012 U.S. average= 29.4 births per 1,000 females age 15-19

SOURCE: CDC National Vital Statistics Reports, "Births: Final Data for 2012", 62(9)2013. [6]

It's not just teens having accidental pregnancies either. In Texas, more than half of **all** pregnancies (54%) are accidental.[7]

The situation has worsened recently in Texas counties that used to be served by Planned Parenthood. In 2011, Texas defunded Planned Parenthood, leaving many counties without any services.[8] A new study reports that those counties had an increase in Medicaid-covered births in the 18 months following funding removal, whereas counties with services showed a decrease in Medicaid-covered births.[9]

Teenage pregnancy has social consequences. Compared with women who have babies later in life, teenagers who have babies are:

- Less likely to finish high school;
- More likely to rely on public assistance;
- More likely to be poor as adults; and
- More likely to have children who have poorer educational, behavioral, and health outcomes over the course of their lives than do kids born to older parents.[10]

Accidental pregnancies cost the taxpayer too. In 2010, more than 57%[11] of all births in Texas were publicly funded at a cost of nearly $3 billion—almost a third of which was paid by Texas.[12] That is our tax dollars that could be invested in education or health, paying for a preventable situation.

Our country as a whole loses out too, as each student dropping out of school represents about $260,000 in lost earnings, taxes, and productivity.[13]

Pregnancy is not the only unintended consequence of sex—**disease** is another consequence and a potentially fatal one. Texas ranked third among the 50 states in the number of HIV[14] diagnoses in 2015. Texas also ranks 16th in syphilis, 13th in chlamydia, and 11th gonorrhea.[15] In fact, Austin has more sexually transmitted disease cases than 50 other cities surveyed, and Dallas is ninth![16]

The disease risk is higher for young people too. Of the 20 million new sexually transmitted infection or "STI" cases every year, about half in 2000 occurred among individuals aged 15 to 24.[17]

This book aims to improve these statistics, providing marital education in an easy-to-read, nonjudgmental fashion. Why "marital" education instead of "sex" education? We chose this name in hope of reaching parents who support abstinence-only education.

Abstinence-only education may have a positive benefit in delaying the onset of sexual activity[18]—but it can lead to marriage at an earlier age. Without marital education, those young couples may not know how to plan their family. Thus, even if they are married, young parents are still at risk for dropping out of school with all of the negative consequences mentioned above.

Further, although pregnancy is an important focus, the information presented here is also relevant for marriages in which children are not an option. We believe that whether you have children or not, reproductive health care and education is important to your well-being, and that your well-being is important to everyone's well-being.

This book thus provides a basic education in the types of family planning and disease prevention methods available and discusses their failure rates and the common reasons for failure. It makes suggestions for doubling or trebling up (using two or three different methods) to improve the chances of avoiding accidental pregnancy and disease.

Our purpose here is not to scare young people but to provide essential information in a balanced and nonjudgmental way. Hopefully, this book will also be able to connect with parents who have been pro–abstinence-only and encourage them to consider marital education in their communities. In Texas, and other states with high HIV rates, it may mean the difference between a happy healthy life, and a shortened one fighting HIV.

A copy of this book for personal use can be downloaded at www.Treble-Up.com. A $1 donation is suggested per copy for school use. Read it, pass it on, and if you get the opportunity, vote for abstinence-plus–marital education to be taught in your local schools.

Chapter 1. Actual Birth Control Failure Rates

Birth control is not as good as most people think in preventing accidental pregnancies. You may be familiar with numbers quoting failure rates in "perfect" use. But how many users are perfect?

Let's take condoms as an example. Condoms are reported to have perfect use failure rates of 1 to 2%. But how many condoms were always stored perfectly? Have you ever left them in the car? In your wallet? At the bottom of a messy purse? How long did they sit in a hot warehouse before being delivered to your local drugstore? How many people know exactly how and when to use a condom? How many have a perfect fit? How many vaginas are frictionless? How many use the perfect lubricant? Or any lubricant at all?

You can see that there are a lot of ways imperfections can creep in—and they do as reflected by the 13% failure rate.

Even if condom usage is "perfect," one or two women in a hundred will still get pregnant in the first year of using condoms.

So let's look at the actual failure rates of the various forms of birth control, starting from the least effective to the most effective.[19]

Method	Actual Failure Rate (Percent of pregnancies in first year of use)
None	85%
Spermicide	28%
Fertility awareness	24%
Withdrawal	20%[20]
Female condom	21%
Cap	14%
Male condom	13%[21]
Diaphragm/sponge	12%
Pill/patch/ring	9%
Injection	6%
Implant	<1%
Intrauterine device	0.2–0.8%
Tubal ligation	0.5%
Vasectomy	0.15%

If you don't use **any** method of birth control, there is an 85% chance of getting pregnant in the first year.

Spermicides are chemicals that kill sperm. They are inserted into the vagina before intercourse to prevent pregnancy. Spermicide is typically available as a foam or jelly, although other forms are available. While it **can** be used alone, you can see from the 28% failure rate that it isn't very effective by itself. In fact, spermicides are intended to be used **with** barrier methods of birth control, such as the condom, diaphragm, cap, sponge or ring.

Fertility awareness methods are a form of family planning that relies on tracking one's periods and ovulation in various ways and not having sex at those times when it is possible to get pregnant. This method is inexpensive and doesn't have any side effects. Some women choose to use fertility awareness methods for religious reasons. For example, the Catholic church approves of various fertility awareness methods.

However, using fertility awareness methods for birth control requires careful record keeping, diligence, and regular periods. As the chart above shows, they're not very reliable with a 24% failure rate.

We will provide a whole chapter on using this method and each of the other methods later, so let's move on.

Withdrawal means that the male pulls out of the vagina before ejaculation, and it's not very effective by itself either (20% failure rate). It is, however, free and has no side effects—if you don't count pregnancy or disease!

Male and female condoms have a couple of benefits, namely that they are easy to buy and no prescription is needed. They also protect against **both** disease and pregnancy, and these are the **only** methods that do. However, used alone, they are not very reliable, failing 13–21% of users within the first year.

The diaphragm and the sponge are similar to the condom in that they are barrier methods of birth control—physically blocking sperm from reaching an egg, instead of relying on hormones to change egg production.

The sponge is a round piece of white plastic foam that is inserted into the vagina before sex and left in afterwards for 6 hours. The sponge works in two ways: it blocks the cervix to keep sperm from getting into the uterus, and it continuously releases spermicide.

The diaphragm is a Frisbee-shaped rubber cap that fits over the cervix. It is coated with spermicide, inserted into the vagina before sex, and not removed for six hours after sex.

The failure rate is pretty high—12% for both of these barrier methods. The cap is very similar to the diaphragm, but smaller and with a 14% failure rate.

The pill, the patch and the ring are all hormonal methods of birth control. These act by changing the body in various ways. For example, some prevent eggs from being released from the ovaries, others thicken cervical mucus to prevent sperm from entering the uterus, and others thin the lining of the uterus to prevent implantation. The pill is taken every day, the patch is applied weekly, and the ring is inserted into the vagina every month. These each have about a 9% failure rate.

Hormones may have some negative side effects, but they can also have significant positive side effects. In fact, many women take some kind of hormone to regulate their periods and reduce the monthly discomfort. There are also many different kinds of hormonal regimes, and some trial and error may be needed to find one that is suitable for a woman.

The injection is also hormone based and is taken every three months. There is a 6% failure rate for this method. However, one has to go to the clinic every three months to get the shot.

The implant releases hormones from a slender rod inserted under the skin of the arm. It lasts for 3 years, and because no action is required by the user, it is more effective than other methods. Although the Centers for Disease Control and Prevention(CDC) reports a 0.05% failure rate, that is **not** accurate, and many women have complained of unintended pregnancy while using the implant.[22] The manufacturer suggests that when correctly inserted, the failure rate is less than 1%, and that is the number we have used in our chart.[23]

The intrauterine device (IUD) comes in two basic forms—one with hormones and one without. It is inserted into the uterus, leaving small strings protruding into the vaginal canal. The hormonal kind lasts three to five years and the nonhormonal can last ten to twelve years.

The IUD is usually accompanied with some pain on initial insertion, heavier periods for one to three months, and it can be expelled, which is also painful. If your body accepts it, it can be nice to have years of fairly reliable birth control. The failure rate is less than 1%.

The failure rate of the two types of sterilization procedures is also less than 1%. In vasectomies, the vas deferens is cut or tied, and it is usually outpatient surgery, taking about 20 minutes. The man usually takes a couple of days off work. Tubal ligation for a woman is a surgical method, involving anesthesia. Recovery times vary from one to two days to a few weeks. A nonsurgical method was available to women, but has now been taken off the market in the U.S.

Sterilizations are generally not reversible and thus may be appropriate for an older person who already has a family. However, sterilization is also used for medical reasons when pregnancy might be dangerous to a woman's health or when a couple have hereditary problems they do not want to pass on to their children.

Some of you might be surprised that even sterilizations sometimes fail—they do. **No** method is foolproof. We will delve more into the reasons why in chapter 9 on sterilization.

You may have noticed that the failure rate of abstinence is conspicuously absent from our chart. That is because no one has done any research on the topic. Of course, the theoretical use is close to perfect. If you are on a desert island with no other human being present, it may be biologically impossible to get pregnant. However, we are dealing with facts here—not theory. Common sense suggests that in the real world, abstinence as a contraceptive method can and does fail.

For one thing, abstinence is difficult. The sex drive is at its highest when we are young, and it's hard to say no. It can be especially hard when a woman is ovulating because that's when she is most attractive to men.[24]

In addition, abstinence can't work in the event of rape, nor can abstinence from penile-vaginal sex prevent STIs where oral sex and other forms of skin-to-skin contact are occurring. Even if you believe in the power of abstinence-only teaching, remember, women don't always get a choice.[25]

In summary, no method of birth control is perfect, and the very best methods have failure rates of less than 1%. That's still one pregnancy in every hundred or so within the first year of use, and it is something to remember as you consider whether or not to initiate sex in your relationship. Pregnancy is always a risk—married or not.

Further, we only discussed pregnancy as one possible consequence of the failure of birth control. Disease is actually a much **bigger** risk, given that there are 20 million new STI cases in the U.S. every year[26] and only 4 million births.[27]

In the next chapters, we will look at each of these methods more closely, providing instruction on their correct usage, most common reasons for failure, and suggesting ways to triple—treble up—your protection.

If you want to compare the various methods side by side, https://www.bedsider.org/methods has a very convenient graphic that highlights key points as you pass your cursor over each method and also groups methods by feature, such as "most effective" or "hormone free." Additionally, this site is also available in Spanish.

Chapter 2: Fertility Awareness Methods

There are a variety of fertility awareness methods (FAMs) of family planning, but all require that the woman have fairly regular periods and, if not, they will be less reliable. All have the benefit of requiring no medicines or devices—and thus are free from the side effects of medicines or devices. However, they offer no disease protection and have a fairly high failure rate (24%).

Strictly speaking, FAMs are free or nearly so, except for the thermometer needed for temperature-based methods. However, there are various devices that can help with fertility tracking (search "fertility tracking device"), and these can be beneficial. Costs of these devices range from $20 for an ovulation detection test strip to $500 for an electronic temperature-based fertility monitor. There are also phone apps available for tracking fertility, ranging from free to a few hundred dollars or even a monthly subscription fee (search "fertility tracking app").

In general, women are most fertile during the following times:

- 5 days before ovulation
- the day of ovulation
- 12 to 24 hours after ovulation

All fertility awareness methods require that the couple avoid unprotected sex during these fertile times, and the Catholic church teaches abstinence during these times.

However, FAMs can also be used when a couple is ready to have a baby, as it greatly improves a couple's odds of conceiving if sex occurs during the fertile days.

If you are interested in FAM-based family planning, it is generally recommended that you undergo some training in your chosen method. Furthermore, it may be best to start charting your cycle a few months before you get married, so that you have a good baseline with which to start.

Although these methods are somewhat complex, we present some basics here so that you can begin to learn about these methods and have a basis for further investigation.

There are several FAMs available, but the methods are grouped into one of three types: 1) symptom-based methods, 2) calendar-based methods, and 3) breastfeeding-based methods. There are many combination methods as well, using two or more of these various methods.

Symptom-Based Methods

The three primary signs of a woman's fertility are basal body temperature, thickness of the cervical mucus, and the cervical position. Hormones can also be detected, but detection requires the purchase of test kits. Some are marketed for getting pregnant, rather than avoiding it.

Temperature goes up very slightly after ovulation. For temperature-based methods, you must take your temperature orally each morning **before** you get out of bed using a special basal temperature thermometer, which can detect very small changes.

If you record your temperature every day, you will see that prior to ovulation your temperature is somewhat regular. As you approach ovulation, you may notice a slight decline, followed by a sharp increase **after** ovulation.

Because the increase happens after you have ovulated, this method is best used by those who have time to track and study their charts for a few months in advance, to ensure the best chances of success.

Illness, travel, and alcohol or drug use can affect temperature and make it difficult to establish an accurate reading. Lack of sleep can also affect temperature reading, so it is important to get at least three consecutive hours of sleep before taking your basal body temperature.

The mucus-based method tracks mucus quality, which is more wet and slippery during ovulation. To practice this method, collect the mucus from the vaginal opening with your fingers by wiping them from front to back. Record it daily on your fertility calendar by making note of the color, consistency and the feel. Ovulation usually occurs within one to two days of when the mucus is clearest, slippery, and most stretchy, if not on the peak day itself.

With training one can also feel the position of the cervix. Feeling for the position of the cervix is done once a day in the evening. This method is never used alone, but only in conjunction with another fertility indicator such as temperature or mucus.

During the fertile phase the cervix moves upward, away from the vaginal opening. Around the time of the "peak" mucus symptom, at the time of maximum fertility, the cervix reaches its highest point making it difficult to reach with the finger. This is called the maximum cervix position. During the fertile phase the cervix becomes progressively softer and feels wet due to the presence of mucus. The cervical opening will gradually open to admit a fingertip and will be at its maximum diameter at ovulation.

Any change in position and consistency of the cervix from its original infertile state indicates the beginning of the fertile phase and usually corresponds with the beginning of the mucus symptoms.

Calendar-Based Methods

Calendar-based methods determine fertility based on a record of the length of previous menstrual cycles. They include the rhythm method and the standard days method.

Before relying on the rhythm method, a woman records the number of days in each menstrual cycle for at least 6 months. The first day of monthly bleeding is always counted as day 1.

The first day of the fertile time is estimated by subtracting 18 from the length of the shortest recorded cycle. The last day of fertility is estimated by subtracting 11 days from the length of the longest recorded cycle. Unprotected sex is then avoided during this fertile period.

The concept behind the standard days method is that women with regular menstrual cycles lasting 26–32 days can prevent pregnancy by avoiding unprotected intercourse on days 8 through 19. This 12-day fertile window takes into account the variability in the timing of ovulation and the viability of sperm in the woman's reproductive tract. A string of color-coded beads in the shape of a necklace (CycleBeads) helps users of the Standard Days Method to identify the fertile and infertile days of their cycle, as well as to monitor their cycle length.

Breastfeeding-Based Methods

The lactational amenorrhea method (LAM) is a method of avoiding pregnancy based on the natural infertility that occurs after giving birth when a woman is amenorrheic—not having periods—and fully breastfeeding the new baby. The rules of the method help a woman identify and possibly lengthen her infertile period.

A woman can use LAM if:

- her period has not returned since delivery (light spotting during the first 56 days does not count), AND

- she is breastfeeding her baby on demand, both day and night, and **not** feeding other foods or liquids regularly, AND
- her baby is less than six months old.

As you can see, fertility awareness–based methods are somewhat complicated and require some training and consistency. Further, there are many variations on FAMs that are not covered here. Our treatment of this topic is by necessity incomplete, and we only touched on the basics. Really, an entire book could be written on this topic, and many have been.

For a quiz on which FAM might be best for you, visit:

http://iusenfp.com/which-method-of-nfp-is-right-for-me/.

For more information on fertility awareness–based methods, the links below may be helpful:

http://www.usccb.org/issues-and-action/marriage-and-family/natural-family-planning/

https://ccli.org

https://www.plannedparenthood.org/learn/birth-control/fertility-awareness

http://www.flowersfertility.com

http://holistichormonalhealth.com/difference-between-fam-methods/

Chapter 3: Withdrawal

Withdrawal is a method of birth control wherein a husband withdraws from his wife's vagina before ejaculation, thus avoiding depositing the sperm that can lead to pregnancy. It is not very effective, with a 20% failure rate. However, it can be made better, and it can be combined with other methods of birth control, such as condoms, fertility awareness, diaphrams, and the like.

There is little, if any, research available on why withdrawal fails, but it is suspected that the two main reasons are lack of control and sperm in the urethra.

Younger men in particular may lack the control needed to withdraw each and every time before ejaculation. However, this should improve with age and experience. Be careful to aim well away from your wife's genitals when you do ejaculate, as even small amounts of ejaculate may have unintended consequences. Consider keeping emergency contraception (aka the morning-after pill) in your medicine cabinet, just in case ejaculate gets in or near the vagina. Emergency contraception can prevent pregnancy for up to five days after unprotected sex. See chapter 10.

The other issue is the potential of a few sperm having been left behind in the urethra from a prior ejaculation. Preejaculate, or "precum"—the drop of lubricant that appears at the tip of the penis early in arousal—does not normally contain sperm, but it may pick up any that were left behind as it travels the urethra. You can reduce the possibility of this occurring by being careful to urinate every time before using withdrawal.

One of the nice things about withdrawal is that it's always free and always available. Also, it can be combined with any other method of birth control for improved effectiveness. Unfortunately, withdrawal offers **no** protection against STIs. Still, combined with condoms or other methods of birth control, it can certainly improve your success rate in family planning.

Chapter 4: Spermicides

Spermicides are chemicals that kill sperm. They act by preventing the sperm from reaching the egg. Spermicides are available in different forms, including creams, film, foams, gels, and suppositories.

Spermicides are easy to use, do not require a prescription, and have no effect on a woman's hormones. However, they can be a bit messy and can cause irritation to some users, especially on frequent use. Further, they are not for rectal or oral use.

In addition to being sold at many drugstores, spermicides can be purchased at Amazon.com. The cost is about $10–15 for 10–30 uses.

Spermicides should always be used **with** barrier methods of birth control, such as the condom, diaphragm, cervical cap, and sponge. They are very unreliable by themselves.

Spermicides are not for rectal or oral use, nor for more than once-a-day vaginal use. In fact, there is evidence that spermicide use may **increase** the transmission of HIV because the active ingredient (nonoxynol-9) is a surfactant (a soap), which may irritate sensitive tissue on frequent use, allowing easier entry by HIV.[28] Thus, if your partner has HIV, you should look for a different form of birth control and disease prevention—such as condoms coupled with withdrawal and regular HIV medication.

As with most forms of birth control, spermicides do not reduce the risk of contracting STIs, especially the viral infections. Therefore, if disease transmission is a concern, a male condom or female condom **must** be used as well.

There are condoms that are labeled as having spermicides on them. However, the amount is **insignificant**, and a second spermicide should be used with a condom.[29] In addition, some men find the spermicide in the condom irritating.

Correct spermicide use varies slightly based on the type you buy (film, cream, gel, etc.). For best practices, always follow the instructions on the packaging.

Most forms require you to clean your hands thoroughly with soap and water and then sit or lie down to apply. Then, using a finger or an applicator, gently insert the spermicide deep into the vagina, waiting at least 10 minutes between applying it and having sex. It usually stays effective for one hour after insertion, but you must apply more **each time** you have sex.

It is important that spermicide remain in place at least six to eight hours after intercourse, because the spermicide takes a few hours to completely neutralize the sperm. Therefore, a woman should not douche (rinse the vagina) for six to eight hours after sex.

Chapter 5: Condoms

There are two kinds of condoms, the male condom and the female condom, but storage and lubrication rules are similar for both of them.

Condoms have few side effects, although some people have an allergy to latex. If that is the case, you can switch to a condom made from polyisoprene or polyurethane, although there are fewer studies available on their effectiveness.

The most frequently reported downside of using a latex condom was diminished sensation. However, male condoms are also available in natural fibers (lambskin). These have a much better feel, but are more expensive and a shorter package life. Also, the lambskin condom may be less effective at preventing STIs, although few studies have been done. People who use lambskin often combine the lambskin condom with withdrawal to reduce the risk of disease and pregnancy.

Another option is the female condom or polyurethane condoms. Some men prefer the feel of these over a latex condom because the texture is soft and moist.

One of the benefits of both male and female condoms is that they are available over-the-counter (at Amazon and drugstores) to anyone. They are relatively inexpensive at $2–5 each, the female condom usually costing more than the male condom.

The primary benefit of condoms is that they can prevent or at least reduce the risk of disease transmission and they are the only birth control method that does this. They are not of high reliability though and should be combined with other types of protection, such as spermicides or withdrawal and the pill, implant or IUD.

Storage

Condoms should be stored in a cool, dry place away from any sharp objects and direct sunlight. Don't keep them in your pocket, wallet, car, or bathroom for long periods of time (over one month), because excessive heat, moisture and friction can damage condoms over time.

Instead, make a small kit and store your condoms in a container that protects them from sharp objects, grit, pressure and heat. Since some people can have an allergic reaction to latex or spermicides, you might have a selection of condoms to choose from, including the latex condom, the polyurethane condom, and even the female condom.

The kit can contain other important items, like a water-based lubricant, spermicidal foam or jelly, emergency contraceptives, towelettes, hand sanitizer, nail brush, and the like.

Why a nail brush? It is a good idea to have clean nails before intimate contact, as many germs can be carried under the nails. Even if no STI germs are present, it is easy to cause vaginitis or a urinary tract infection if your hands and nails are not clean.

Since you have to use a new condom **every** time you have sex, it's a good idea to keep a supply in your kit, and keep your kit close by.

Lubrication

Most male and female condoms come prelubricated, but adding extra water-based or silicone lube can make condoms feel better and also help keep them from breaking. It must be a water-based or silicone-based lubricant, not an oil-based lubricant.

Never use petroleum jelly (Vaseline), lotion, baby oil, butter, or cooking oils on latex or polyisoprene. The oil damages the material and may make condoms break more easily.

To use a lubricant, put a few drops on the outside of the male condom once you're wearing it. If needed, add some during sex too. For the female condom, add a bit to the inside before putting it in the vagina, or add more to the penis during sex.

Practice makes perfect, so it's a good idea to get used to putting on either the male or the female condoms before you actually use one.

Manufacturing Defects

Even if you store, lubricate and use the condom correctly, sometimes a batch of condoms is recalled due to manufacturing problems. Condoms made overseas may be more prone to manufacturing error, since we have standardized testing of condoms in the U.S. If you wonder if your condom was any good, test your condom after you use it by filling it with water. If it leaks, use an emergency contraceptive. See chapter 10.

Using the Male Condom

Always check the expiration date, and make sure there aren't holes in the packaging before opening the condom—you should be able to feel a little air bubble when you squeeze the wrapper. If a condom is torn, dry, stiff, or sticky, throw it away.

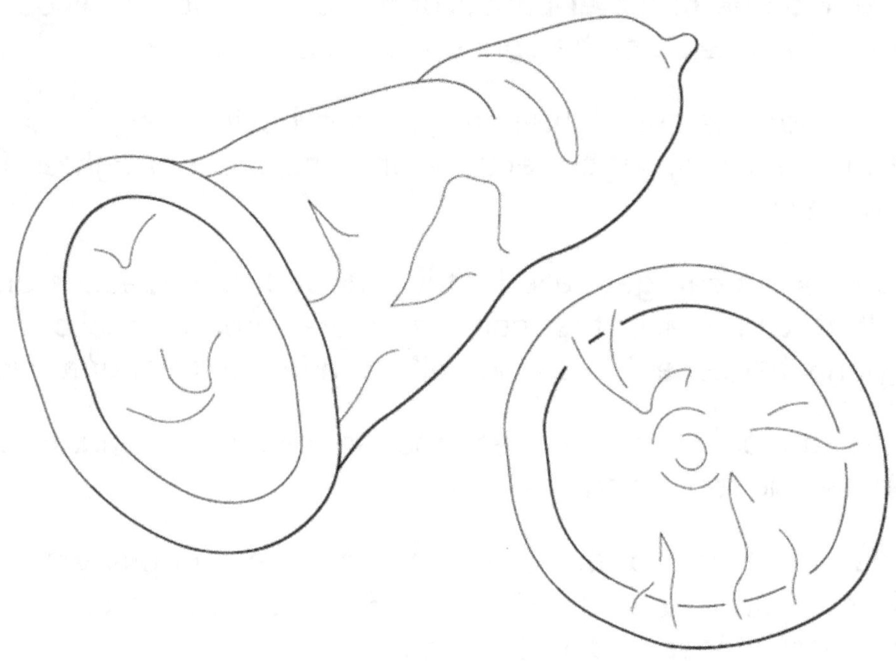

Unrolled (left) and rolled (right) condoms.[30]

Be careful in opening a new package. Don't tear the condom with your teeth, scissors, jewelry or other sharp objects.

Roll the condom on when your penis is erect (hard), but BEFORE it touches your partner's mouth or genital area (vulva, vagina, anus, buttocks, and upper thighs)—and wear it the **whole** time you're having sex.

This helps protect you from many STIs that are transmitted through skin-to-skin touching. It also prevents contact with preejaculate, which can have STI germs and may contain some sperm.

Make sure the condom is ready to roll on the right way: the rolled rim should be on the **outside** so it will unroll easily. If you accidentally put a condom on inside out, do NOT flip it around and reuse it—get a new one.

If you're uncircumcised, pull your foreskin back **before** placing the condom on the tip of your penis.

Squeeze the tip of the condom between your thumb and finger, and place it on the head of your penis. The little bit of space at the top is needed to collect semen (cum) and needs to be empty of air.

Unroll the condom down the shaft of your penis all the way to the base.

You can put a few drops of water-based or silicone lubricant inside the tip of the condom and/or on the outside of the condom once it's on.

If you feel the condom getting tighter as you are having sex, it may be about to break. Pull out and reposition it correctly. Condoms can get tighter if your partner squeezes on the way in.

By contrast, the condom can get pulled off if your partner squeezes on the way out. Another thing that can make the condom more prone to slip is use on the uncircumcised penis because the foreskin allows a fair amount of motion.

Be careful and try to feel for each of these movements happening. If it does, pull out as described below and reposition the condom.

After you ejaculate take hold of the rim of the condom and pull your penis and the condom out of your partner's body. Do this BEFORE your penis goes soft, so the condom doesn't get too loose and let semen out.

Carefully take off the condom away from your partner so you don't accidentally spill semen. Throw the condom away in the garbage—don't flush it down the toilet (it can clog pipes). Wash your hands and penis with soap and water.

You **cannot** reuse condoms. Use a new condom every time you have vaginal or other sex. You should also use a new condom if you switch from one kind of sex to another.

Sometimes people are afraid to ask for condom use because they are embarrassed to ask, or they worry it suggests that their partner has a disease. However, frank discussions about protection are an important part of intimacy.

It's easy to make condoms fun and sexy—all it takes is a little creativity, confidence and a positive attitude! Protect yourselves from pregnancy and/or STIs so you can both relax and focus on the intimacy.

Lastly, you may recall that the actual failure rate of condoms is 13%, which is pretty high. You should always combine condom use with other forms of birth control, such as a spermicide or withdrawal and the pill, implant or IUD.

IF THE CONDOM BREAKS, SLIPS or LEAKS, use an emergency contraceptive. See chapter 10.

Using the Female Condom

The female condom is the only woman-controlled method that reduces the risk of transmission of STIs. It is available over the counter and can be inserted ahead of time to avoid interruption during sex. One nice advantage is that it can be used during menstruation. However, it is less reliable than the male condom and certainly less discreet than other methods since part of the condom hangs out of the vagina. It may also cause some discomfort or irritation, and it can make noise.

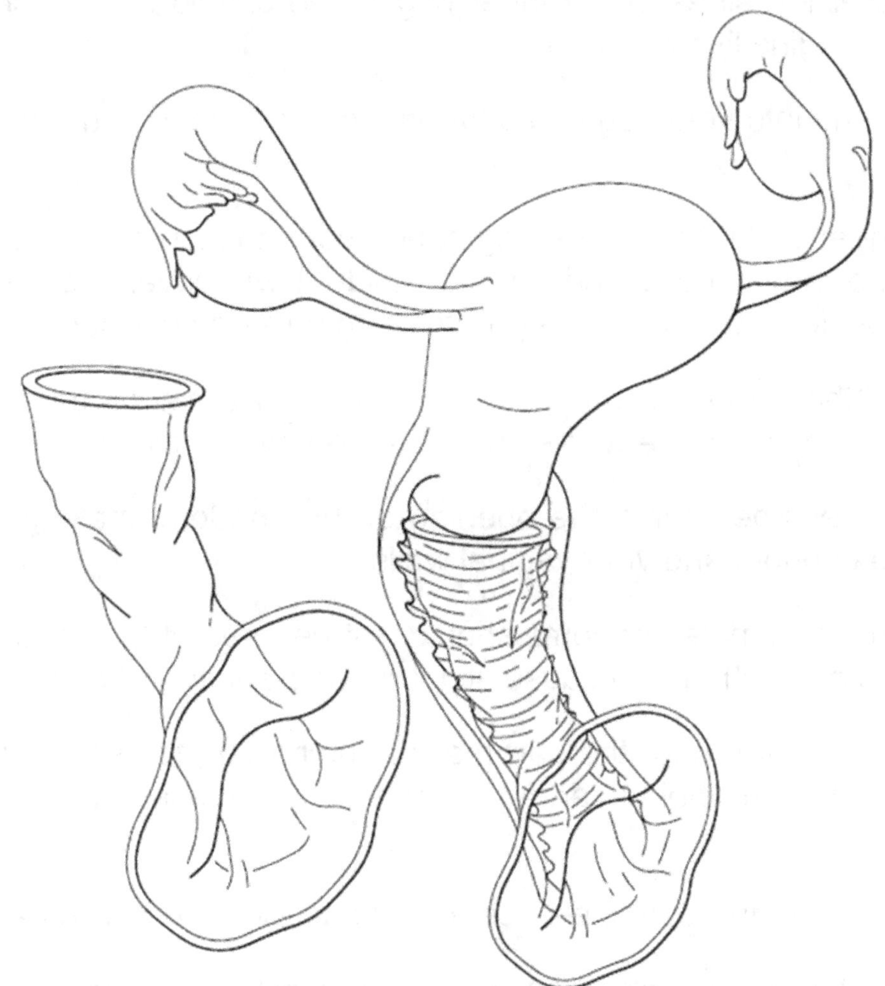

Female condom (left) inside the vagina covering the cervix (right).[31]

That said, sometimes men prefer the female condom more than the male condom because they say it offers more sensation. Thus, men should try one and if they like it, include a few in their kits.

The female condom is bigger than a male condom, but it's not uncomfortable if inserted correctly. If you can use a tampon, you can probably use a female condom.

Check the expiration date on the package, and then open it carefully.

The female condom comes already lubricated, but you can add more lube to the inside if you want. You can also put spermicide or lubricant on the outside of the closed end before insertion.

Relax and get into a comfortable position. Standing with one foot on a chair, lying down, or sitting are common positions—kind of like how you'd put in a tampon.

Squeeze together the sides of the inner ring at the closed end of the condom and slide it into your vagina like a tampon.

Push the inner ring into your vagina as far as it can go, up to your cervix. Make sure it's not twisted.

Pull out your finger and let the outer ring hang about an inch outside the vagina. The large ring at the open end of the female condom will cover the area around the vaginal opening—it is normal for this part to hang outside your body.

You can insert the female condom up to eight hours before sex. Like the male condom, it should be used the whole time you are having sex.

Guide your partner's penis into the opening of the condom, making sure it doesn't go between the condom and your vaginal walls.

Female condoms and male condoms should **not** be used at the same time because they can stick to each other and cause slippage or breakage of one or both devices.

After sex, twist the outer ring (the part that's hanging out) to keep semen inside the pouch. Gently pull it out, being careful not to spill any semen. Throw it away in the trash (don't flush it).

Female condoms are not reusable—use a new one every time you have sex.

Slippage of the female condom can occur, especially if the penis is large, sex is vigorous, or if you are inexperienced at using it.

If it slips, stop immediately! Take the female condom out carefully, so that the sperm stays inside the pouch. Use a new female condom if you continue having sexual intercourse. Add extra lubricant to the opening of the pouch or on the penis and then insert the new female condom.

Remember the female condom isn't very reliable by itself (21% failure rate). Always combine it with other forms of protection, such as spermicide or withdrawal plus the pill, implant or IUD.

Some drugstores, such as Walgreens, carry female condoms, but they are not as easy to find as male condoms. Ordering online (Amazon) is a great option, or you may be able to find a clinic nearby that has them.

Remember, both sexes can use male or female condoms—the name only relates to **where** it is used—not who buys it and makes it available.

IF THE CONDOM BREAKS, SLIPS or LEAKS, use an emergency contraceptive. See chapter 10.

Chapter 6: Female Barrier Methods

There are a number of barrier methods that are used by females in addition to the female condom we just covered. Each is based on physically blocking the sperm from reaching the egg, and each is intended to be used only with spermicides. These include the diaphragm, the sponge, and the cervical cap.

If any of these barrier methods fail (e.g., by slippage), use an emergency contraceptive. See chapter 10.

Diaphragm

The diaphragm is a shallow, dome-shaped cup made of silicone. It is used with spermicide and inserted into the vagina, where it covers the cervix and keeps sperm away from the egg.

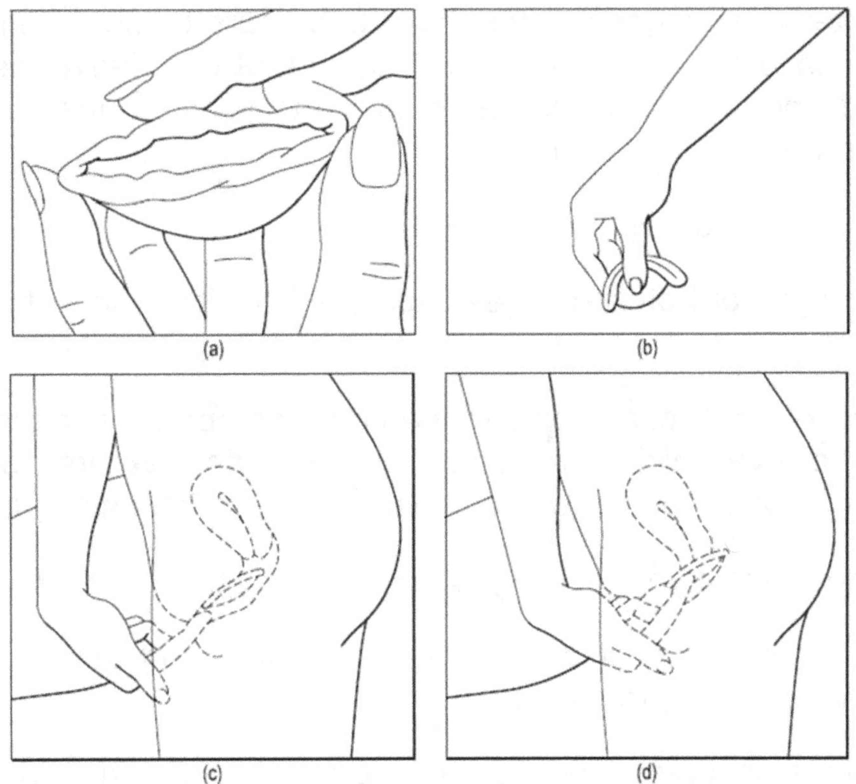

Spermicide added to diaphragm (a), folded in half (b) inserted into vagina (c) and pushed deep to ensure it sits over the cervix (d).[32]

It has several advantages, namely that it can be used hours before sex, it doesn't affect a woman's hormones, and it is very discreet. However, you do need a prescription, and you have to use it each and every time. It can be tricky to get in or out, and if you react badly to either the spermicide or the silicon, you may not be able to use the diaphragm.

In addition, it can be pushed out of place by large penises, vigorous sex, or certain positions, and it won't prevent disease transmission. Finally, some women find they get frequent urinary tract infections while using a diaphragm.

The failure rate of the diaphragm is 12%, but it can be higher if you have already had a child.

At full price, the diaphragm can cost as much as $90, and some clinics may charge for a fitting fee. However, it may be covered by health insurance or Medicaid, and clinics may offer them for reduced cost or even free. Further, with proper care, a diaphragm can last for years, making it very cost-effective in the long run.

A diaphragm can be inserted just before sex, but it can also go in hours before as well. But no matter when it goes in, you have to be sure to leave it in for at least six hours **after** you have sex. If you have sex again that day, leave the diaphragm in place, and add more spermicide deep in your vagina. Just don't leave the diaphragm in for more than 24 hours.

To use it, wash your hands with soap and water.

Check the diaphragm for holes and weak spots. Fill it with water—if it leaks, throw it away.

Put a tablespoon or so of spermicide in the cup, and spread some around the rim, too. Any kind of spermicide foam or gel will do, except for the film or insert/suppository types. Don't forget to check the expiration date of the spermicide.

Either sit or lie down, as if you're going to put in a tampon.

Separate the outer lips of your vagina with one hand, and use the other hand to pinch the rim of the diaphragm and fold it in half.

Put your index finger in the middle of the fold to get a good, firm grip. Yes—you may touch the spermicide.

Push the diaphragm as far up and back into your vagina as you can, and make sure to cover your cervix.

Leave in for at least six hours after sex, but no more than 24.

If you have sex a second time, leave the diaphragm in place and insert more spermicide. Start the six-hour clock again.

When the six hours have passed, remove the diaphragm. Again, wash your hands with soap and water. Put your index finger inside your vagina and hook it over the top of the rim of the diaphragm. This can be a bit of a stretch. Pull the diaphragm down and out.

If you have trouble with removing the diaphragm, ask your doctor about getting an inserter, or consider switching to another method.

Finally, take good care of your diaphragm and it can last for several years. After you take it out, wash it with mild soap and warm water and allow to air dry. Do **not** use with powders or oil-based lubricants (like Vaseline or cold cream) or silicon-based lubricants.

Cervical Cap

A cervical cap is a silicone cup that covers the cervix to keep sperm out of the uterus. It is similar to the diaphragm, but smaller. Shape varies, but some cervical caps (e.g., the FemCap) have a shape like a sailor's cap, but with a brim that is bigger on one side. The spermicide fits into the bowl, and is also used on the other side, between the brim and the dome. Because of the snug fit, there is no need to add spermicide each time you have sex.

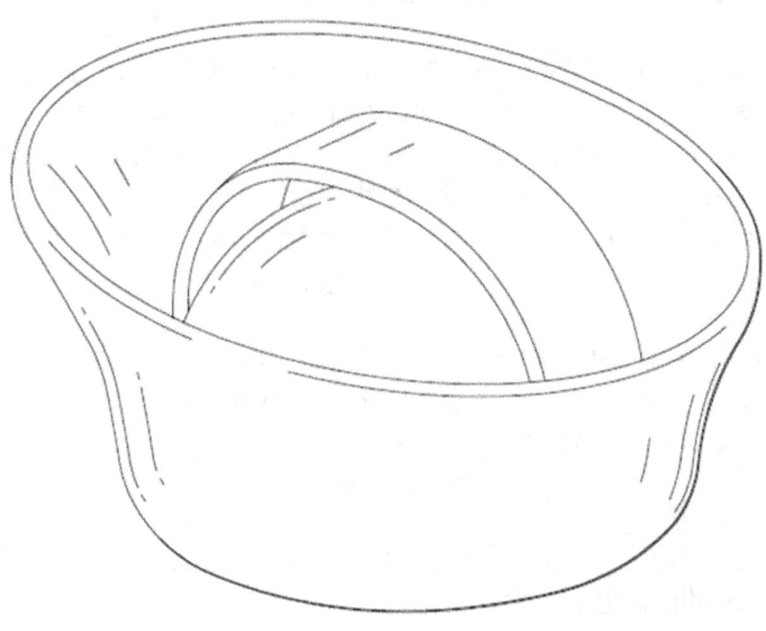

Cervical cap.[33]

Cervical caps are much less commonly used than diaphragms—they're mainly for women who, because of the shape of their vaginas, find it difficult to keep a diaphragm in place.

The retail cost of the cap is about the same as the diaphragm ($90), and clinics may also charge for the exam or a fitting fee. However, it may be covered by health insurance or Medicaid, and clinics may offer it at reduced cost or even free.

It has advantages and disadvantages similar to those of the diaphragm and sponge, but there are some differences. It doesn't affect your hormones. You can put it in hours in advance, and you can have sex as many times as you like while it's in without adding more spermicide. It can be left in place for up to 48 hours. Neither you nor your partner should be able to feel it.

However, it can be tricky to get in and out, and it causes irritation, allergies or urinary tract infections in some women. You have to use it every time you have sex, and it offers no protection against STIs. Plus, it can get pushed out of place by large penises, vigorous sex, or certain sexual positions. As with the other barrier methods, it is more effective if you have never had children (14% failure rate[34]).

To use it, first wash your hands with soap and water (as always). Check the cervical cap for holes and weak spots by filling it with water. If it leaks, throw it away. Put a quarter teaspoon or so of spermicide in the bowl, and spread some around the rim, too. Flip it over to the side with the removal strap and put another half teaspoon in the indentation between the brim and the dome.

Sit or lie down, like you're going to put in a tampon. Put your index and middle fingers into your vagina and feel for your cervix, so you'll know where to place the cap. Separate the outer lips of your vagina with one hand, and use the other hand to squeeze the rim of the cap together. Slide the cap in dome and strap side down with the long brim being inserted first. Push down toward your anus, and then push up and onto your cervix. Make sure your cervix is totally covered.

Leave in for at least six hours after sex. To remove it, again wash your hands with soap and water. Put a finger inside your vagina, get a hold of the removal strap, and rotate the cap. Push on the dome a bit with your finger to break the suction. Hook your finger under the strap and pull the cap out.

The cap can last up to two years if you take good care of it. Wash it with mild soap and warm water and allow to air dry.

Don't use powders or oil- or silicon-based lubricants on your cap.

Sponge

The sponge is a round piece of white plastic foam with a little dimple on one side and a nylon loop across the top that looks like shoelace material. It's pretty small—just two inches across—and it is inserted into the vagina before sex. The sponge works in two ways: it blocks the cervix to keep sperm from getting into the uterus, and it continuously releases spermicide.

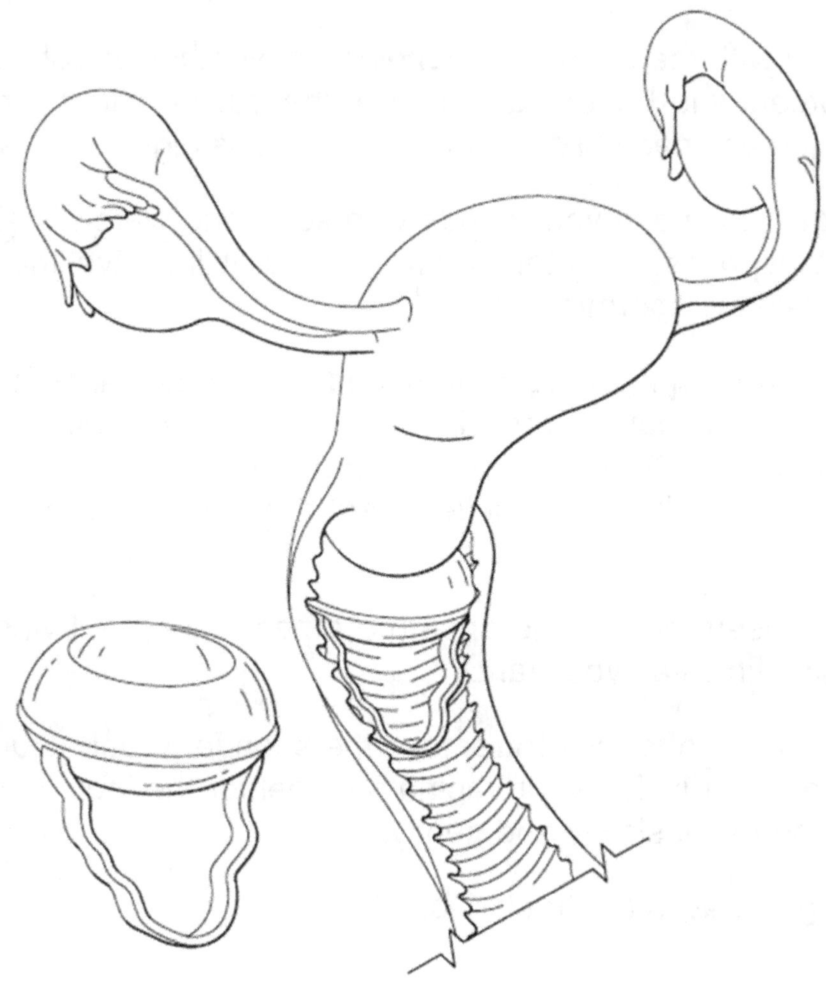

Sponge (left) fitted into vagina over cervix (right).[35]

The sponge has several advantages. It can be used up to 24 hours in advance, and you can have sex as many times as you like while it's in. Neither you nor your partner should be able to feel the sponge. It doesn't affect your hormones, and no prescription is necessary.

However, some women have a hard time inserting it, it can cause irritation, and it may make sex messier or even drier. Some women are allergic to the sponge itself or to the spermicide and can't use the sponge.

The sponge is cost-effective, costing $3–8 each, but one sponge can last up to 24 hours, no matter how many times you have sex. It can be bought online (Amazon, CVS) and in some drug stores, and your local family planning clinics may offer free or low-cost sponges as well.

Failure rates vary with the sponge depending on whether or not you've already had a child. For women who haven't given birth, the actual failure rate is 12%, but for women who've already had children, the failure rate is higher.

To use a sponge, first wash your hands with soap and water. Wet the sponge with at least two tablespoons of water before you put it in. Give the sponge a gentle squeeze to activate the spermicide.

With the dimple side facing up, fold the sponge in half upward. Slide the sponge as far into your vagina as your fingers will reach. The sponge will unfold and cover the cervix when you let go. Slide your finger around the edge of the sponge to make sure it's in place. You should be able to feel the nylon loop on the bottom of the sponge.

You should only insert the sponge once (no repeat uses), but when it's in, you can have sex as many times as you want.

Wait at least six hours after sex to remove the sponge. Wash your hands with soap and water. Put a finger inside your vagina and feel for the loop. Once you've got the loop, pull the sponge out slowly and gently.

Throw the sponge away in the trash. Don't flush it!

Chapter 7: Hormonal Methods

To date, there are no male hormone–based methods of birth control, but scientists are working on one. In fact, a male hormonal method is being clinically tested in India. However, it will be some time yet before such methods are available in the U.S.

However, there are many hormone-based options available for women, and they include combination estrogen and progestin pills, progestin-only pills, and the patch, the ring, the injection, the implant and the hormonal IUD. We will cover the hormonal IUD in chapter 8 on IUDs.

Combined hormone methods work by suppressing ovulation and thickening cervical mucus, while progestin-only methods reduce the frequency of ovulation and rely more heavily on changes in cervical mucus and thinning the uterine lining.

The hormone-based methods are reversible, and once you stop using them, you should again be fertile, although with longer lasting methods, it can take longer for fertility to return.

Reasons for Failure

For any method of birth control that requires daily use or use with every instance of sex, the primary cause of failure is user error. Thus, the pill most often fails because the woman forgets to take it or fails to take the pill at about the same time each and every day. The patch, shot and implant are somewhat more effective, because they last longer and present fewer opportunities to forget.

Another cause of failure is that unless started within five days of your period, they take at least a week to become effective.

Other causes of failure include inflammatory bowel disease or other digestive disorders. These can interfere with the absorbance of the pill, making it less effective because it didn't reach the body. This problem only applies to the pills, which are the only oral forms of hormonal birth control.

Certain medications also interfere with all hormone-based methods of birth control, including certain seizure or migraine meds, St. John's wort, certain antibiotics (rifampicin and rifabutin) and certain HIV drugs (protease inhibitors [PIs] and nonnucleoside reverse-transcriptase inhibitors [NNRTIs]).

Occasionally there are also manufacturing errors—pills, the ring, the patch, the shot or the implant—are released with insufficient drug or even with just placebo or with some other manufacturing defect. Most recently, millions of Gildess pills were recalled due to a decreased level of drug.[36]

Side Effects

Because hormones do change the body, a prescription is required for their use. These are drugs, and as drugs there may be unintended side effects. In some cases the side effects are severe enough to prevent the use of hormones.

Common side effects include mood changes, spotting between periods, reduced or missed periods, breast tenderness, nausea and vomiting, change in weight, and a change in libido. More serious but rare risks include blood clots. Some cancers are at increased risk, while others are at decreased risk.

However, many women do not experience significant problems, and potential side effects include regular and lighter periods and less premenstrual syndrome (PMS).[37] In fact, the pill is often prescribed to treat awful periods.

It is important to discuss your medical condition with your doctor so that the best regime can be selected for you at your age. For example, smokers over age 35 have increased risks for certain side effects, and some believe that hormone-based methods may not be suitable for the young who have yet to establish a mature functional fertility system. Also, it may be necessary to do a little trial and error to get the best dosage for you. If hormones don't agree with you, you should consider fertility awareness–based methods, barrier methods, or an IUD.

This description of side effects is by no means comprehensive, but the following web pages will provide more information:

https://www.bedsider.org/features/819-combined-hormonal-versus-progestin-only-birth-control

http://www.healthline.com/health/birth-control-effects-on-body

Ultimately though, you should discuss potential side effects with a medical professional as this is a complicated topic and everyone is different.

Access

Some states have written laws that allow pills and patches to be sold over the counter, allowing the pharmacist to write the prescription. Oregon, California, and Washington, DC, have such laws, and similar laws are pending in other states. Another law that makes access easier is one that allows the pharmacist to provide 12 months of pills at once. To see what's available in your state visit:

https://fivethirtyeight.com/features/some-states-are-making-it-easier-to-get-birth-control/ or https://freethepill.org.

In some states you may not be able to access birth control that requires a prescription without parental permission. Texas is like that. However, Title X clinics will provide teen access, and the nearest Texas clinic can be found at https://www.whfpt.org/find-a-clinic.

In addition, new companies are being launched to provide mail-order prescriptions and delivery. Check out Nurx (which delivers in Texas), Maven or Lemonaid or search "online prescription birth control."

The Pill

A prescription is needed for the pill in the U.S., and once you have one you can receive mail-order refills. The cost varies up to $50 per month, plus any examination costs. Health insurance will usually pay for pills, and reduced cost or even free pills may be available at clinics.

Whichever pill you take, you have to remember to take it every day at about the same time, which is one of its main disadvantages. There are apps that will remind you to take a pill, but missing pills or taking pills late is a frequent cause of failure (9% failure rate).

Thus, longer acting forms of hormone-based birth control typically have better failure rates because the user has fewer opportunities to forget its application. Don't forget to use a backup for seven days if you don't start within five days of your period or if you forget or are late with a pill.

Patch

The patch is a thin, beige piece of plastic that looks like a square Band-Aid. It's a little less than two inches across, and only comes in the one color. It costs about the same as the pill and has the same side effects, but, in addition, the adhesive may also cause irritation. It has a 9% failure rate.

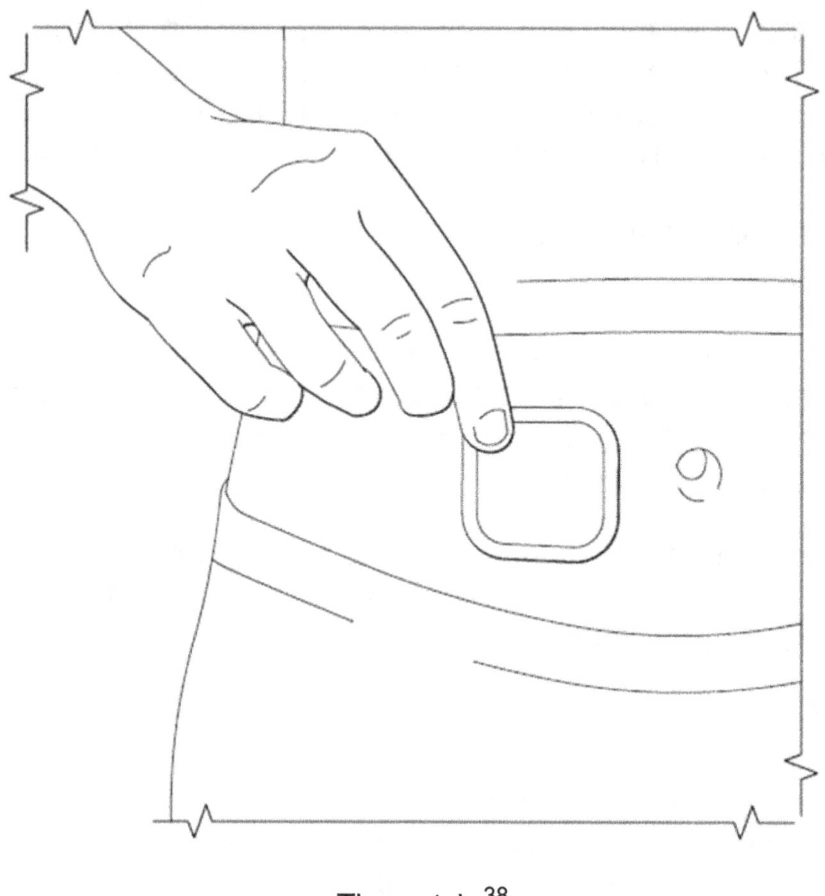

The patch.[38]

The patch is stuck onto clean skin where it releases hormones that prevent the ovaries from releasing eggs. The hormones also thicken the cervical mucus, helping to block sperm from reaching the egg.

It is applied once a week, every week on the same day for three weeks, and thus it is less likely to be forgotten or late. Then you skip a week.

To use it, pick a patch change day.

You'll probably get your period during the patchless week, and you may still be bleeding when it's time to put the patch back on. That's normal.

You can also continue using patches, changing them once a week without taking a break. For most people this will mean that their period will not come. Some will have spotting after a few months—this is normal.

If you start the patch within the first five days of your period, you're protected from pregnancy right away. If you start later, you'll have to wait seven days before you're protected and use a backup method.

Carefully consider where you want the patch—it'll be there for a full week. What will you be wearing? Are there any skin folds there? Can you easily check that it has not fallen off?

Don't use body lotion, oil, powder, creamy soaps (like Dove or Caress) or makeup on the spot where you put your patch. These can keep the patch from sticking.

Only peel off half of the clear plastic at first, so you'll have a nonsticky side to hold. Don't touch the sticky part of the patch with your fingers.

Apply it and press the patch down for a full 10 seconds to get a good, firm stick.

Check your patch every day to make sure it's sticking right.

When you take a patch off, fold it in half and throw it in the trash.

If you want to skip a period, just skip the week off and add a new patch in the fourth week.

If your patch falls off, but it has been less than 24 hours, you can just reattach the same patch in the same location (as long as it is still sticky). You can also replace it with a new patch.

If your patch has fallen off for more than 24 hours, you MUST apply a new patch (throw out the one that has fallen off). The day that you replace the patch will then become the new day of the week that you change your patch (so if you replace a patch on a Tuesday, then you will change it on Tuesday of the following week).

You should also use a backup birth control method for the first seven days after you have applied a new patch, because it had been more than 24 hours since the previous patch fell off.

Ring

The ring is inserted into the vagina to surround the cervix. It is discreet, and a new ring is inserted every three to four weeks. Don't forget to use a backup for 7 days if you don't start within 5 days of your period.

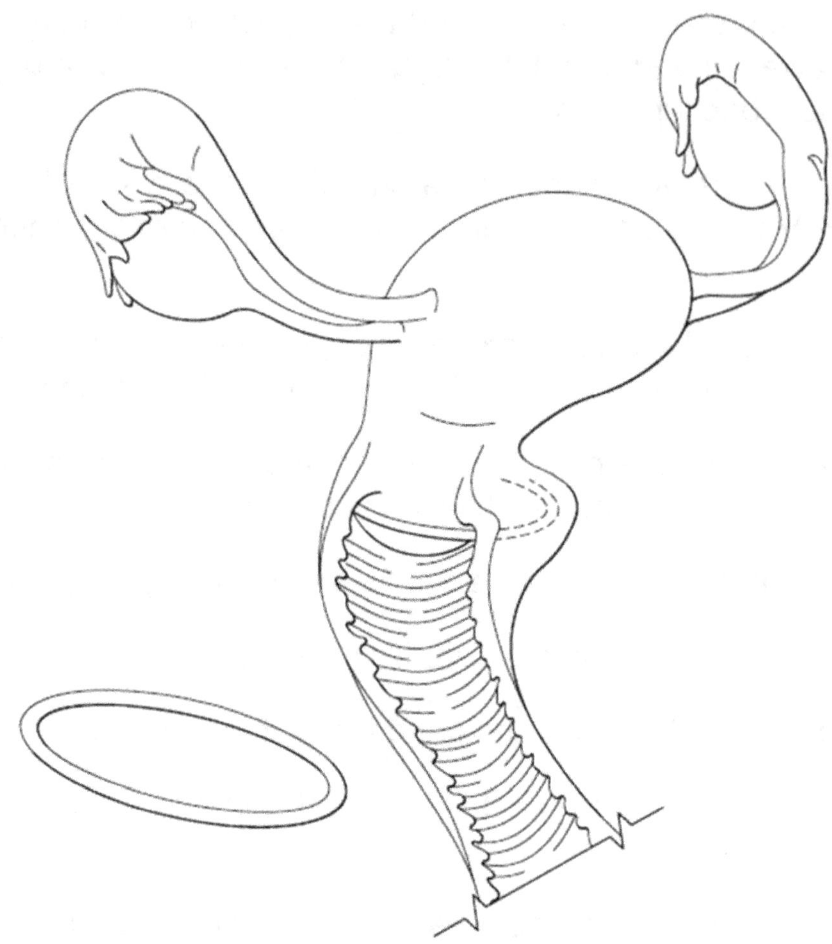

Ring (left) fitted into vagina over cervix (right).[39]

If you have health insurance or Medicaid, the ring may be free or it may be available at reduced cost at some clinics. Otherwise, the ring averages around $55 a month.

The ring may have all the side effects of any hormone-based method of birth control. However, the ring uses a lower dose of hormones than other methods, so there may be fewer negative side effects. Your partner typically won't feel anything, although some do. In clinical studies 90% of partners did not find this to be a problem.

To use it, wash your hands with soap and water. Remove the ring, squish it between your thumb and index finger, and insert it like a tampon. Keep the resealable pouch for disposing of the used ring.

The exact position doesn't really matter, as long as you're comfortable.

Once you insert the ring, leave it in for three weeks. Take it out for the fourth week. Then insert a new ring and start the cycle again.

To take the ring out, wash your hands with soap and water. Insert your finger into the vagina and feel for the ring. It can be a bit of a stretch. Hook your finger on the lower edge and pull. Dispose of it by resealing it in the pouch and putting the pouch in the trash.

When the ring is out, you'll probably get your period. If you're still bleeding when it's time to put the ring back in, don't worry. That's totally normal.

If you want to skip your period, don't do the week off. Just insert a new ring at 3 weeks.

The ring sometimes does come out, especially if a tampon catches on it. If this happens, wash it and reinsert it. If it breaks, use a new one.

If the ring has been out of your vagina for more than three continuous hours, use a backup method of birth control for the rest of the month.

Don't use the ring with the diaphragm as the ring may interfere with the fit of the diaphragm.

Shot

The shot is just what it sounds like—a shot that keeps you from getting pregnant—and is called Depo, Depo-Provera, or DMPA (depot medroxyprogesterone acetate). Once you get it, your birth control is covered for three full months—there's nothing else you have to do. It is reversible, but may take longer since it's intended to last longer. It has a 6% failure rate.

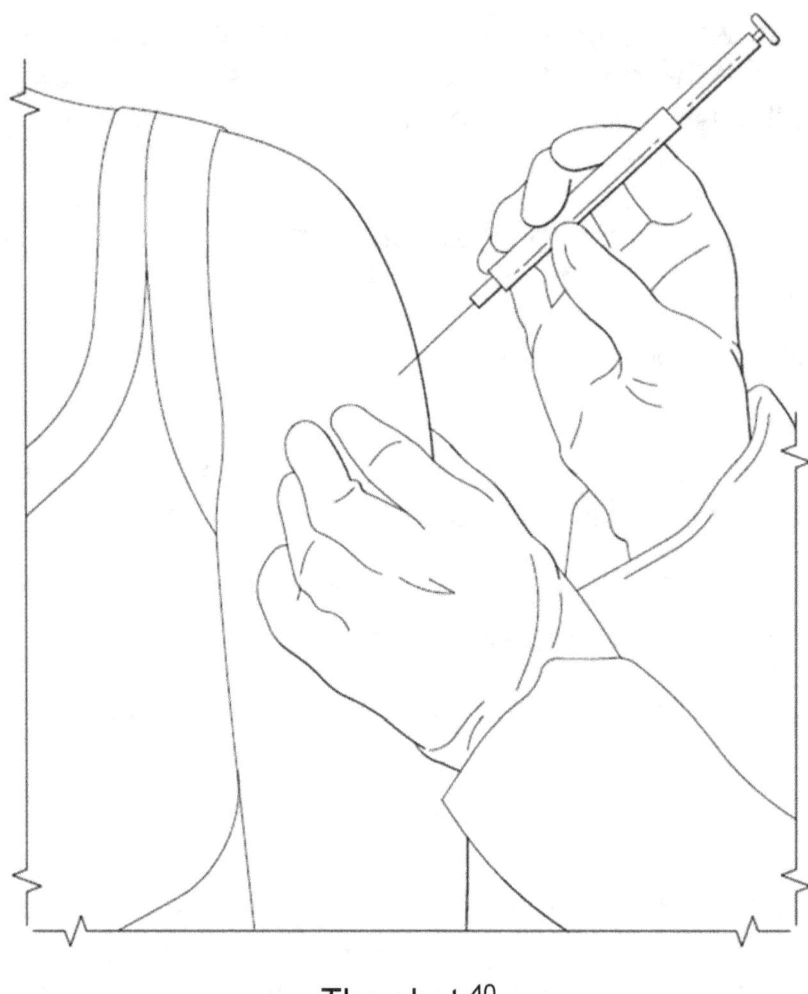

The shot.[40]

It costs about $45–$100, but if you average it over the three months it's not too expensive. It is only available at clinics with a prescription.

The advantage is that it is very discreet—no one can tell if you have taken the shot. The disadvantage is that you have to go to the clinic and get the injection. There is also the minor pain of getting an injection.

Because you only need to remember four times a year to get it, it's less prone to failure by forgetting. If you miss a shot, however, you increase the risk of getting pregnant. Use a backup method until you get the next shot.

If you start the shot within the first 5 days of your period, you're protected from pregnancy right away. If you start later, you'll need to use a backup method for 7 days.

There is one at-home option called SubQ Depo. This is a progestin-only shot that is injected into the skin. Of course, then you have to inject yourself, but some people are able to do this. If you are interested in this option, the prefilled syringe can be purchased at pharmacies with a prescription, and your doctor or nurse can teach you how to do the injection.

Implant

The implant (Nexplanon) is a matchstick-size rod that's inserted under the skin of the upper arm. It is discreet, but may be visible in some women, especially thinner women.

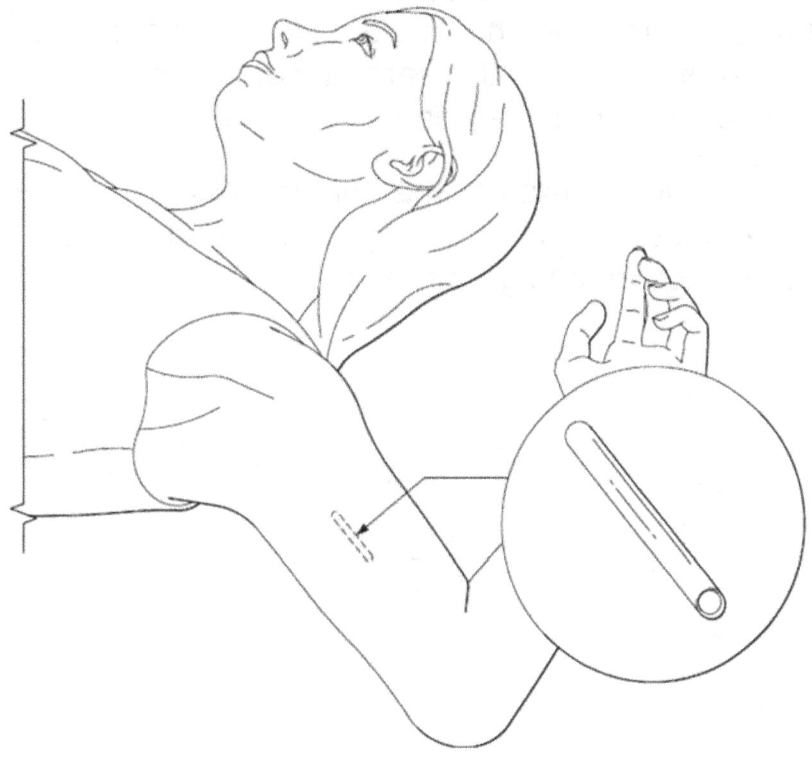

The implant.[41]

The implant releases progestin, preventing the ovaries from releasing eggs, and also thickening cervical mucus, which helps block sperm from reaching the egg. It prevents pregnancy for up to three years and thus is known as a long-acting, reversible contraceptive (LARC), and because it requires no action after insertion, its failure rate is below 1%. As with other hormonal methods, it is effective right away if started within five days of your period; otherwise, use backup for a week.

It's expensive, at $800–900, but averaged over the length of use, it's not bad ($300/year or $25/month). It's also covered by health insurance and Medicaid, and it may be available at lower cost at clinics.

Of course, you need a prescription, and it is inserted into the arm at the clinic. The doctor will numb a small area of your upper arm with a painkiller and then insert the implant under the skin.

You should be able to feel the implant under your skin, and you should check regularly to make sure it stays in place. There may be pain and bruising at the site, and some women report menstrual bleeding for some time until they adjust.

When it's time to take the implant out, your doctor will numb your arm again, make a tiny cut in your skin, and remove the implant. If you want to continue using the implant, you can get another one at the same time. There may be a charge ($300) to remove the implant as well, or it may be free.

Because there is nothing for you to do, the implant may be the most reliable of the purely hormone-based methods with an actual failure rate of less than 1%. But it's not perfect, and women sometimes get pregnant while using it.

Chapter 8: Intrauterine Devices

The intrauterine device, or IUD, is a small, often T-shaped birth control device that is inserted into a woman's uterus to prevent pregnancy. Like the implant, an IUD is a LARC.

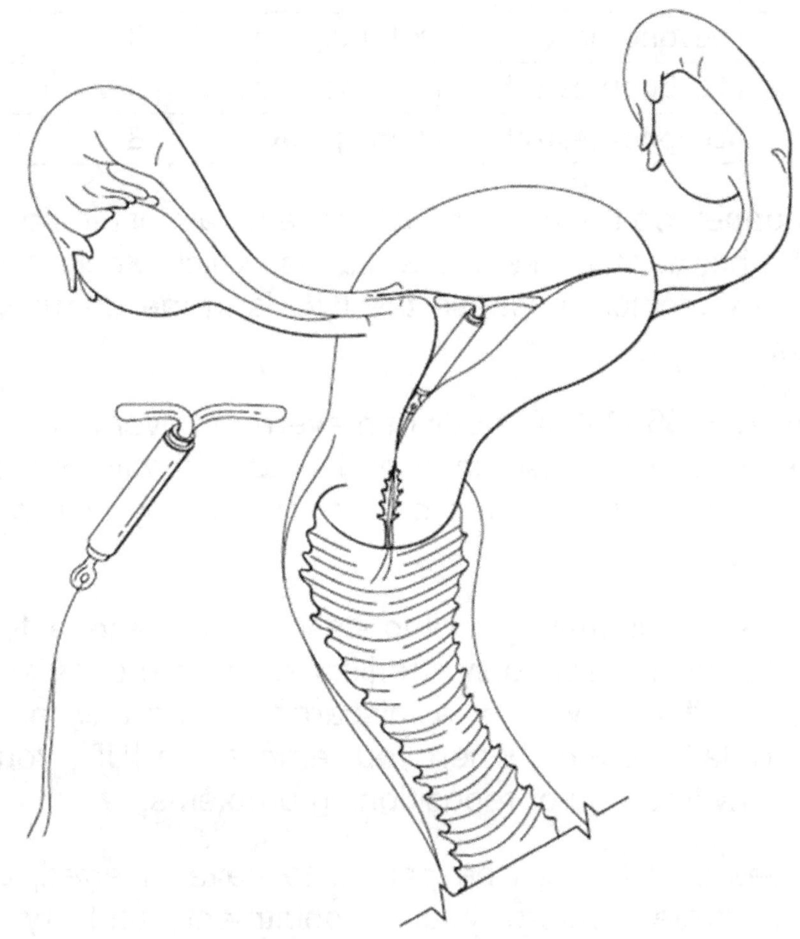

Intrauterine device (right) inserted into the uterus (right).[42]

There are two basic kinds—the copper IUD and the hormonal IUD, which is a progestin-only device. The copper IUD can last for up to 10–12 years, and the hormonal one lasts from three to seven years.

Name	Active Agent	Dose	Approval Duration (years)
ParaGard	Copper	—	10–12
Mirena	Levonorgestrel	20 mcg/day	5–7
Liletta	Levonorgestrel	18.6 mcg/day	3–5
Kyleena	Levonorgestrel	17.5 mcg/day	5
Skyla	Levonorgestrel	14 mcg/day	3

Sperm don't like copper, so the copper IUD makes it almost impossible for sperm to get to the egg. The hormone thickens the mucus, which blocks the sperm and also reduces ovulation. In addition, because the IUD is in the uterus, the rare fertilized egg cannot implant.

The cost seems high at $500–900, but when averaged over three to twelve years of service, it is quite affordable. Insurance and Medicaid will usually pay for it, and lower costs may be available at some clinics. There may also be a charge for its removal.

The advantage of the IUD is that it is completely discreet and lasts a very long time, making it fairly reliable. In fact, only sterilization is more reliable. IUDs can be inserted immediately after delivery or a miscarriage, and they are often used after the first birth control failure. Plus, when you remove the IUD, you should return to full fertility, barring any infection or repositioning problems.

However, both types of IUDs can be painful to have inserted, causing cramping afterward. Take ibuprofen before your appointment, and try to schedule the appointment when you're on your period or ovulating. Even if there is some pain for a few days, it might be worth it for years of less than 1% failure rate protection.

You may also find that the first few periods are harder. However, the hormonal IUDs may reduce menstrual bleeding or stop menstruation altogether.

The most serious complication associated with IUDs is infection. They sometimes are expelled and they can sometimes puncture the uterus, both of which are painful and can lead to infection. Most clinics will schedule a visit at one month to make sure that everything is OK.

The procedure is in the beginning similar to getting a Pap smear. You'll put your feet in stirrups. The doctor will put the IUD in a small tube that she'll insert into your vagina and then through the cervix into the uterus. Then she'll push the IUD out of the tube and pull the tube out. Strings attached to the IUD will hang one to two inches into the vaginal canal, but these are not visible and will barely be noticeable. The strings are there so that the IUD can be removed.

Check the string from time to time, especially for the first three to six months to make sure it stays in place.

Wash your hands with soap and water, then sit or lie down.

Put your finger in your vagina until you touch your cervix, which will feel firm and rubbery like a small ball.

Feel for the strings. They should be neither longer, nor shorter than usual, and you should not feel the hard part of the IUD. If any of these occur, go to the clinic right away.

Other signs of a possible problem are severe cramping, a sudden increase in pain, heavy or abnormal bleeding, an abnormal discharge or a fever.

You should be concerned if all of a sudden sexual intercourse hurts. This may be an indication your IUD has moved. It could be sticking out of your cervix just enough to make the area tender.

Don't tug on the strings! If you do, the IUD could move out of place.

Although the IUD sounds a bit scary, most gynecologists and family planning practitioners use them. In fact, one study showed that use of IUDs by female ob-gyns is three times greater than that of the general public.[43] This suggests that they are safer than the average person thinks.

Chapter 9: Sterilization

Sterilization is a surgical procedure to prevent pregnancy and is chosen when your family is complete, when pregnancy is medically dangerous, or when parents have genetic problems they don't wish to pass on to their children. It may also be chosen by younger people who are **certain** they do not want children, but there is a lower incidence of regret when a person is older (> 30 years).

Generally speaking, for women the tubes are blocked or cut, so the egg can never reach the uterus. For men, the vas deferens are blocked or cut, so the sperm never reach the ejaculate. Sterilization is generally not reversible, and it provides the best protection of any form of birth control.

That said, it isn't perfect, and pregnancies sometimes happen with either form of sterilization. Further, there are several different techniques that can be used, and some are more effective than others.

Some of the reasons for failure include medical error. There are occasions when the physician blocked only one tube and forgot the other. Sometimes the wrong tubes are tied. Similar errors also occur in vasectomies—the vas deferens is very small and easily missed.

Another failure mode is failure of the blockage, and sperm or eggs still get through tiny channels. However, the most common error for failure of vasectomy is failure within the first three months because sterility is **not** immediate. It takes some time for all the sperm to clear out.

Generally speaking, the advantages of sterilization are that it is hormone free, permanent and discreet. Further, since all you are doing is blocking the tubes, there should be no change in your body, sex drive, or periods.

The disadvantage is that the method requires some intervention inside your body, and therefore there will be some pain. There can be complications from any surgical procedure. Also, sterilization does NOT protect against STIs, including HIV.

For more information on sterilization, see:

https://www.uptodate.com/contents/permanent-sterilization-procedures-for-women-beyond-the-basics

http://www.uptodate.com/contents/vasectomy-beyond-the-basics?source=search_result&search=vasectomy&selectedTitle=3%7E29

Sterilization is covered by most health insurance and Medicaid, and it may be offered at a reduced price at certain clinics. At full price, sterilization for women can cost from $500 to $5,000 and a vasectomy can cost as much as $1,000. For a lifetime of use, that's a pretty good price.

Tubal Ligation for Women

In tubal ligation, the fallopian tubes are blocked with a ring or burned or clipped shut. Portions of the tube can even be removed. This procedure is typically performed with the patient under general anesthesia in a hospital. It can be done by laparoscopy or a mini-laparotomy.

For a laparoscopy, the surgeon makes a small incision through the abdomen and inserts a laparoscope to view the pelvic region and tubes. He or she then closes the tubes using clips, tubal rings or electrocoagulation (using an electric current to cauterize and destroy a portion of the tube).

The patient can usually go home the same day and resume intercourse as soon as it's comfortable. Risks include pain, bleeding, infection and other postsurgical complications, as well as an ectopic pregnancy—in which an egg implants in the tubes instead of in the uterus.

During a mini-laparotomy, the surgeon makes a small incision (about two inches long) and ties and cuts the tubes without the use of a viewing instrument. In general, mini-laparotomy is a good choice for women who undergo sterilization right after childbirth. Patients usually need a few days to recover and can resume intercourse after consulting with their doctors.

Often tubal ligation is done immediately after birth, especially C-section births, since the woman is already in the hospital and undergoing surgery. This option has the advantage of being very discreet.

Vasectomy for Men

During a vasectomy, the testicles and scrotum are cleaned with an antiseptic and possibly shaved. You may also be given an oral or intravenous medicine to reduce anxiety and make you sleepy.

The vas deferens is located by touch. A local anesthetic is injected into the area.

Your doctor makes one or two small openings in the scrotum. Through an opening, the two vas deferens tubes are cut. The two ends of the vas deferens are tied, stitched, or sealed. Electrocautery may be used to seal the ends with heat. Scar tissue from the surgery helps block the tubes.

The vas deferens is then replaced inside the scrotum and the skin is closed with stitches that dissolve and do not have to be removed.

The procedure takes about 20 to 30 minutes and can be done in an office or clinic. It may be done by a primary care physician, a urologist, or a general surgeon.

A no-scalpel vasectomy is also available. This method uses a small clamp with pointed ends. Instead of using a scalpel to cut the skin, the clamp is poked through the skin of the scrotum and then opened. The benefits of this procedure include less bleeding, a smaller hole in the skin, and fewer complications. The no-scalpel vasectomy is as effective as traditional vasectomy.

If you are interested in sterilization, talk to your doctor about the pros and cons of the various methods available before you decide which type of procedure to use.

Chapter 10: Emergency Contraception

Sometimes people aren't given a choice about whether or not to have sex. If you are female and are raped, there are some contraceptives designed for just that situation.

Emergency contraception is birth control that prevents pregnancy after sex, which is why it is sometimes called "the morning-after pill," "the day-after pill," or "morning-after contraception." It is appropriate to use in cases of rape, or in cases in which a condom breaks or slips off during use or when a pill was forgotten.

The name is a bit misleading—you don't have to wait until the morning after. You can use emergency contraception right away or up to five days later.

Emergency contraception makes it much less likely you will get pregnant. But emergency contraceptives are **not** as effective as other forms of birth control, like the pill, implant or IUDs. So, if you are sexually active or planning to be, do not use emergency contraception as your only protection against pregnancy.

In addition, emergency contraception does not protect against sexually transmitted infections—only condoms do.

Your options for emergency contraception include:

- emergency contraceptive pills (also called "morning-after pills") and
- the copper T IUD

Three types of emergency contraceptive pills are available: combined estrogen and progestin pills, progestin-only pills, and antiprogestin pills.

Pills combining estrogen and progestin are no longer available as dedicated emergency contraceptive pills in the U.S., but certain regular combined oral contraceptive pills may be used as emergency contraceptive pills. However, you should consult with a medical practitioner to determine the correct timing and dosage, as this varies by brand. The Princeton University web page at https://ec.princeton.edu/questions/dose.html#dose also has information on this topic.

In the U.S., progestin-only emergency contraception is available over the counter (e.g., at Amazon or a drug store) without age restrictions to either women or men. Look for Plan B One-Step, Take Action, Next Choice One Dose, My Way or other generic versions in the family planning aisle.

Antiprogestin pills may also be available outside the U.S., but inside the U.S., a prescription is needed.

A common side effect of emergency contraceptive pills is nausea and vomiting. If you experience vomiting within three hours of taking one, contact your physician or pharmacist right away. Another dose may be recommended.

The copper T is an IUD that a trained clinician inserts into the uterus up to five days after sex to prevent pregnancy. The copper T IUD does not affect ovulation, but it can prevent sperm from fertilizing an egg. It may also prevent implantation of a fertilized egg.

 As emergency contraception, the copper T IUD is much more effective than emergency contraceptive pills, because it reduces the risk of getting pregnant by more than 99%, whereas the morning after pills are only 88% effective. Another advantage to the copper T IUD is that you can keep it in place to prevent pregnancy for up to ten or twelve years.

If you have pelvic inflammatory disease (PID) or an active gonorrhea or *Chlamydia trachomatis* infection, IUD insertion is not recommended. However, if you have an asymptomatic gonorrhea or chlamydia infection, IUD insertion is considered safe.

For more information on emergency contraception, visit: http://ec.princeton.edu/emergency-contraception.html.

Pregnancy is only one risk of rape—disease is another risk that applies to both women and men who are raped. If you are raped, you should visit a medical practitioner and consider a course of treatment against bacterial infections.

Preventive treatment for gonorrhea, chlamydia, and trichomonas infections usually includes three antibiotics. Some are taken once, while others are taken one to three times daily for 7, 10 or 14 days, depending on the antibiotic.

Preventive treatment for HIV may also be recommended, but must be initiated early. Your medical practitioner will not only discuss the potential risks of getting HIV and the risks of treating it with antiviral therapy, but also recommend a course of action.

The risk of contracting HIV will vary for vaginal versus anal rape, whether or not the skin was torn and whether or not there were multiple assailants. The CDC recommends preventive treatment if the mouth, vagina, anus, or nonintact skin (e.g., a cut) was exposed to the assailant's blood or bodily fluids.

Preventive treatment for hepatitis B may not be needed if you were previously vaccinated, but if not, one vaccine dose is given immediately, followed by additional doses one and six months later.

We know that it will be difficult to share your story with a medical practitioner, but avoiding STIs and pregnancy are worth the effort. Whether or not you tell the police or prosecute is another matter, but at least get medical care and counseling to help you with this traumatic event.

For more information, visit:

https://www.uptodate.com/contents/care-after-sexual-assault-beyond-the-basics.

The Rape, Abuse and Incest National Network can help you locate counseling and support services near you. The network also provides hotlines, which are very helpful in rural areas where clinics may be very sparse. See https://centers.rainn.org.

Chapter 11: Sexually Transmitted Infections

The first edition of this book was incomplete without a chapter on sexually transmitted infections (STIs), a shortcoming this second edition allows us to amend. But don't worry—there will be no gruesome pictures—just some basic information.

The Texas Education Code states that "abstinence from sexual activity, if used consistently and correctly, is the only method that is 100 percent effective in preventing . . . sexually transmitted diseases."[44] This suggests that people may have some misunderstandings about what STIs are and how they can be transmitted. So, let's start there.

An older term for STI that is still in use today is *STD* for *sexually transmitted disease.* However, a significant portion of people with infections do **not** show signs of disease. In fact, about **half** of the people with STIs are without symptoms. Thus, the preferred modern term is *STI* for *sexually transmitted infection,* although STD is still in common use. An even older term is *venereal disease* or *VD* for short.

An STI is any infection that is **primarily** transmitted by sexual activities. However, STIs can be, and often are, transmitted by ways other than intercourse.[45] To name a few of the many methods of transmitting an STI, we know that STIs can be transmitted by kissing; skin-to-skin contact; intimate contact other than coitus; by shared needles; and by exposure to blood, breast milk, and other bodily fluids. Babies can even be born with an STI.[46] In fact, after a period of decline, there has been a recent sharp increase in the number of babies born with congenital syphilis[47] in the U.S.[48]

STIs are **much** more common than people realize. In fact, the CDC estimates about 20 million new cases are detected each year, and about 110 million people, including new and persistent cases, are living with STIs overall.[49] That's **one in three** Americans with an STI!

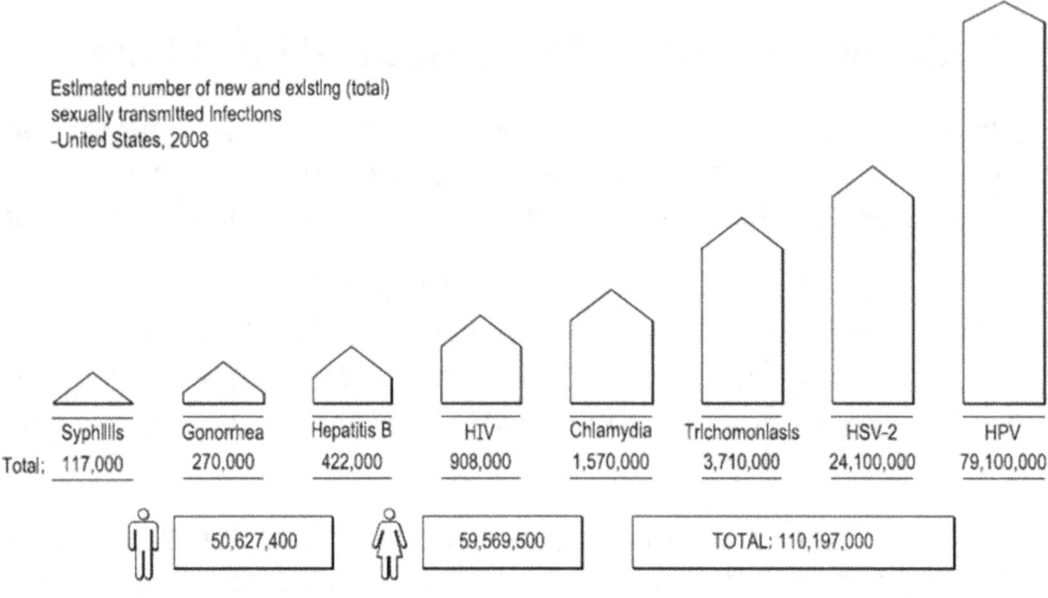

STI incidence in the USA.[50]

The chart above shows that the most common STI is HPV (human papilloma virus), with almost 80 million cases in the U.S. The good news is that there is an effective HPV vaccine, which both members of a couple should get well before marriage.

Genital herpes (HSV-2, or herpes simplex virus–2) is the next most common and is the poster child for why one should use condoms: herpes infections never go away, and the painful virus can be activated whenever the host experiences stress. HSV-1 (oral herpes, also called "cold sores") is also quite common, with about 65% of Americans carrying the virus.[51] Worldwide, about 90% of people have one or both viruses.[52]

There are four main classes of STIs—parasitical, protozoan, bacterial, and viral. We will briefly cover each in turn. Because about half of all STI infections don't show any signs of disease, we are not going to present a list of symptoms for each. Instead, in addition to covering the four main classes, we refer you to the charts below[53] and suggest that **testing** is better than assuming you are disease free because of the absence of symptoms or the state of virginity.

	GENITAL HERPES	**SYPHILIS**
WHAT IS IT	A viral infection of the genital areas and/or mouth.	An infection caused by bacteria that can spread throughout the body.
US INFECTIONS	An estimated 1 million new infections each year, with about 45 million people already infected.	About 46,000 new cases reported each year.
SYMPTOMS	Most people have **no** symptoms. Herpes 1 typically causes cold sores and fever blisters on the mouth and Herpes 2 on the genitals, but, they can infect either area. A herpes outbreak can start as red bumps and then turn into painful blisters or sores. During the first outbreak, it can also lead to flu-like symptoms (like a fever, headaches, and swollen glands).	Symptoms vary based on the course (timing) of infection-beginning with a single, painless sore (called a chancre) on the genitals, anus, or mouth. Other symptoms may appear up to 6 months after the first sore has disappeared including a rash. However, there may be no noticeable symptoms until syphilis has progressed to more serious problems (see below).
HOW IT SPREADS	Through vaginal, oral, or anal sex. It can also be passed through skin-to-skin sexual contact, kissing, and from mother to child during childbirth.	Through vaginal, oral, or anal sex. It can also be passed through kissing if there is a lesion (sore) on the mouth, and from mother to child during childbirth.
TREATMENT	There is **no cure** for herpes-the virus stays in the body and may cause recurrent outbreaks. Medications can help treat symptoms, reduce the frequency of outbreaks, and reduce the likelihood of spreading it.	Antibiotic treatment can cure syphilis, but can't undo damage already done. Both partners must be treated and avoid sexual contact until the sores are completely healed.
CONSEQUENCES IF UNTREATED	Increased risk for other STDs, including HIV. Some people with herpes may get recurrent sores. Passing herpes from mother to newborn is rare, but an infant with herpes can become very ill and even die.	Increased risk for other STDs, including HIV. Untreated, the symptoms will disappear, but the infection stays in the body and can cause damage and even death. Syphilis in women can seriously harm a developing fetus during pregnancy.

	HEPATITUS B VIRUS (HBV)	HIV
WHAT IS IT	A viral infection affecting the liver – HBV can be acute (mild illness lasting for a short time) or chronic (a serious life-long illness)	The human immunodeficiency virus (HIV) is the virus that causes AIDS.
US INFECTIONS	An estimated 40,000 new cases each year (most acquired through sex). Up to 1.2 million people are already infected with chronic HBV.	About 56,000 new infections each year, with an estimated 1.1 million Americans already living with HIV.
SYMPTOMS	Many people don't have any symptoms, especially adults. Tiredness, aches, nausea & vomiting, loss of appetite, darkening of urine, tenderness in the stomach, or yellowing of the skin and the whites of the eyes (called jaundice). Symptoms of acute HBV may appear 1 to 6 months after exposure. Symptoms of chronic HBV can take up to 30 years to appear, although liver damage can occur silently.	Symptoms usually related to infections and cancers people get due to a weakened immune system. On average it takes about 10 years from initial HIV infection to develop AIDS.
HOW IT SPREADS	Through vaginal, oral, or anal sex. Also, through childbirth if the baby does not get vaccinated against HBV; sharing contaminated needles or razors; or exposure to the blood, bodily fluids or saliva of an infected person.	Through vaginal, oral, or anal sex. Also by sharing contaminated needles or drug works; and from mother-to-child during pregnancy or breast-feeding. The chance of getting it through kissing is very low unless there are mouth ulcers.
TREATMENT	Most often, acute HBV is treated with rest, eating well, and lots of fluids. Chronic HBV is treated through close monitoring by a doctor and antiviral medications.	There is **no cure** for HIV or AIDS. Anti-retroviral treatment can slow the progression of HIV disease and delay the onset of AIDS. Early diagnosis and treatment can improve a person's chances of living a longer, healthy life.
CONSEQUENCES IF UNTREATED	Increased risk for other STDs, including HIV. Chronic, persistent inflammation of the liver and later cirrhosis of cancer of the liver. Babies born to infected women are likely to develop chronic HBV infection if not immunized at birth.	Increased risk of other life-threatening infections and certain cancers. Left untreated, HIV infection is fatal.

	GONORRHEA	GENITAL HUMAN PAPILLOMAVIRUS (HPV)
WHAT IS IT	A bacterial infection of the genital areas.	A viral infection with over 40 types that can infect the genital areas, including types that cause warts and cancer.
US INFECTIONS	About 820,000 new cases reported each year. The highest rates are among women aged 20 to 24 and men aged 20 to 24.	An estimated 14 million new cases each year, with at least 79 million Americans already infected. There are vaccines to prevent HPV infections and these are given to teens before they become sexually active.
SYMPTOMS	Most infected people have no symptoms. For those who do, it can cause a burning sensation while urinating, abnormal white, green, and/or yellowish discharge. Women may also have abnormal vaginal bleeding and/or pelvic pain. Men may also have painful or swollen testicles.	Most infected people have no symptoms. But some HPV types can cause genital warts – small bumps in and around the genitals (vagina, vulva, penis, testicles, and anus, etc.). If they do occur, warts may appear within weeks or months of having sex with an infected partner. Cancer-causing HPV types do not cause symptoms until the cancer is advanced.
HOW IT SPREADS	Through vaginal, oral, or anal sex. It can also be passed on from mother to child during childbirth.	Through vaginal, oral, or anal sex. It can also be passed on during skin-to-skin sexual contact, and from mother to child during childbirth.
TREATMENT	Oral antibiotics can cure the infection. Both partners must be treated at the same time to prevent passing the infection back and forth. Both partners should avoid sex until the infection is gone.	There is **no cure** for HPV (a virus), but in most cases, the virus goes away on its own. If the virus does not go away, there are ways to treat HPV-related problems. For example, warts can be removed, frozen off, or treated through topical medicines. Even after treatment, the virus can remain and cause recurrences (warts come back).
CONSEQUENCES IF UNTREATED	Increased risk for infection of other STDs, including HIV. In women, gonorrhea can cause pelvic inflammatory disease (PID) which can lead to infertility or tubal (ectopic) pregnancy. Men may develop epididymitis, a painful condition which can lead to infertility. Babies born to infected women can develop eye infections.	Genital warts will not turn into cancer over time, even if they are not treated. Babies born to women with genital warts can develop warts in the throat. Cancer-causing HPV types can cause cervical cancer & other less common cancers (like anal cancer) if the infection lasts for years.

	CHLAMYDIA	TRICHOMONIASIS (TRICH)
WHAT IS IT	A bacterial infection of the genital areas.	A parasitic infection of the genital areas.
US INFECTIONS	About 1.4 million new cases reported each year. The highest rates are among adolescent women.	An estimated 1 million new cases each year.
SYMPTOMS	Often there are no symptoms. For women who do experience symptoms, they may have abnormal vaginal discharge, bleeding (not their period), and/or burning and pain during urination. Men may have discharge or pain during urination, and/or burning or itching around the opening of the penis.	Often there are no symptoms. Women may notice a frothy, smelly, yellowish-green vaginal discharge, and/or genital area discomfort. Men may temporarily have a discharge from the penis, slight burning after urination or ejaculation, and/or an irritation in the penis.
HOW IT SPREADS	Through vaginal, oral, or anal sex. It can also be passed on from mother to child during childbirth.	Through vaginal sex.
TREATMENT	Oral antibiotics cure the infection. Both partners must be treated at the same time to prevent passing the infection back and forth. Both partners should avoid sex until the infection is gone.	Antibiotics can cure the infection. Both partners must be treated at the same time to prevent passing the infection back and forth. Both partners should avoid sex until the infection is gone. It is common for this infection to recur.
CONSEQUENCES IF UNTREATED	Increased risk for infection of other STDs, including HIV. In women, chlamydia can cause pelvic inflammatory disease (PID) which can lead to infertility or tubal (ectopic) pregnancy. Men may develop pain and swelling in the testicles, although this is rare. Babies born to infected women can develop eye or lung infections.	Increased risk for infection of other STDs, including HIV. Can cause complications during pregnancy.

Parasitical infections, such as public lice (crabs) and scabies, are easily transmitted, even by sharing towels, brushes and clothing. However, they are treatable and not permanent if treated. Small bites or itchiness in the groin area indicate a possible infection, as do small dots on the hair. Scabies can be difficult to detect, but any clinic can check for you.

There are over-the-counter treatments for parasites—but ordinary soap and water and treatments for head lice will not work. Some prescription and over-the-counter treatments kill both the live lice and their eggs (also called nits). Other products require two applications, approximately seven to nine days apart. Check the label to see if the product kills both lice and eggs, and determine how to use it correctly. Your partner should also be treated.

Typically, all your clothes and bedding must also be washed in very hot soapy water and dried with heat. Items that cannot be washed can be placed in a sealed bag for 2 weeks, until the lice and their eggs die out. You can also vacuum rugs and furniture. You don't need to call an exterminator or fumigate your home.

Protozoan infections include trichomoniasis, which is another type of parasite. Trichomoniasis is the most common curable STI. In the United States, an estimated 3.7 million people have the infection. However, only about 30% develop any symptoms. It is treated with prescription medication, and your partner must be treated too.

Bacterial infections, such as syphilis, gonorrhea, and chlamydia, are curable with antibiotics. Get tested and treated, and be sure to follow through on all medication. Make sure your partner gets tested and treated as well. Although curable with diligent treatment, some bacterial STIs can be very serious if untreated or if passed from mother to newborn baby.

Less common bacterial infections include chancroid and lymphogranuloma venereum (LGV). Secondary infections include vaginitis and pelvic inflammatory disease, although these can be caused by other factors too.

Viral STIs, such as herpes, hepatitis, HPV, and HIV, are caused by viruses and many are **not** curable, although they may lie dormant for periods of time. The viral STIs have the worst reputation of all the STIs. HIV will eventually cause AIDS and has killed many people, although it is now treatable, and its progression slowed. HPV can cause cancer. Hepatitis causes liver damage, causes liver cancer and can cause death. Herpes is a lifetime infection, albeit treatable. As with the other STIs, the viral infections are much more serious in the newborn, and it is best to be tested and treated **before** starting a family.

There are discreet lab services available that will test for a complete panel of STIs and provide quick results. Search "STI testing" or "STD testing." You should also be aware that many communities offer free or subsidized STI testing. Check www.freeSTDcheck.org to find a clinic near you.

For more information, see your doctor or visit either of the following sites:

http://www.ashasexualhealth.org/stdsstis/

https://www.plannedparenthood.org/learn/stds-hiv-safer-sex

Chapter 12: Treble-Up

If you have read the previous chapters with some care, we hope you are getting the message that for improved protection it is better to double up or treble up—use two or three forms of birth control. Using more than one method at a time provides overlapping and complementary protection and greatly improves your chances of avoiding an accidental pregnancy and disease.

A man, for example, can use condoms plus a spermicide or withdrawal. For a woman, condoms plus a LARC may offer the best option.

Even if you use only FAMs (fertility-awareness methods), you can combine the temperature method with the mucus method and with test sticks for hormones that coincide with ovulation. Withdrawal might be a good option too. An electronic device to keep track of it all will also improve your chances of success with FAMs.

Methods that typically cannot be combined are those methods that use the same space, such as male and female condoms, the diaphragm and ring, or different types of IUDs. Also, the various hormonal methods should not be combined.

As you can see there are many contraceptive options to choose from, and if you include FAMs in your arsenal of protection, you can even use different methods at different times.

Unfortunately, we don't have very good studies on the actual failure rates of various combined methods of birth control. There are mathematical predictions of effectiveness,[54] but we would like to see actual failure studies rather than theory.

Also, some people suggest that doubling up will do. That may suffice if your only concern is pregnancy, but STIs are a concern too. While pregnancy is well handled by a LARC, such as the implant or IUD, it offers **no** protection against STIs. That is why we suggest the simple message: "Treble up."

A few things to keep in mind as you make these decisions is that **only** condoms protect against disease, and that while all barrier methods should be used with spermicide, spermicides cannot be used too often. Furthermore, some methods cannot be combined, including the male and female condom, the ring and diaphragm, the different IUDs, or different hormone-based methods.

If you are a newlywed couple, and you both practiced abstinence before marriage, do you **still** need condoms to protect against STIs?

Probably, yes—unless you **test** first to confirm there are no STIs.

STIs can be passed through other nonintercourse intimate contacts, and some are passed through needle use. Even babies can be born with HIV or STIs. Further, many STIs can be present without showing any symptoms, and you or your new spouse may not realize there is an infection if there are no symptoms.

It is a good idea to have a full panel of tests, including an HIV test, before marriage, and test for HIV again after the HIV window has passed. The HIV window is a period of time after exposure when HIV cannot yet be detected, and the length of the window varies with the sensitivity of the test. If you and your spouse pass both tests, and neither of you is stepping out, it is probably safe to discontinue condom use.

Another wise precaution is to obtain vaccines before marriage. Right now, the HPV and hepatitis vaccines are available, and in the future, more vaccines will become available. Someday there may even be an HIV vaccine.

We also encourage you to have a contraceptive kit to protect your contraceptives and ensure that you are prepared for any emergency. A man's kit should contain:

- a strong protective and discreet case
- condoms (male or female or both)
- spermicide
- water-based lubricant
- emergency contraceptive pills
- hand sanitizer
- towelettes
- nail brush

A woman's kit can contain the same things, plus whichever of the ring, pill, patch, sponge, cap or diaphragm she is using, unless a LARC (implant or IUD) is being used.

Remember, **treble up: use three forms of birth control** to give you the best in family planning and disease protection.

Final Thoughts

The type of sex education that should be taught in the U.S. has been a major topic of debate and will probably continue to be contentious for years to come.

Some people believe that teaching young people about contraceptives encourages both initiating sexual activity early and having numerous partners. Thus, there has been considerable funding support for abstinence-only education from federal and state governments.

However, the data suggest that abstinence-only is not the best type of sex ed, and Texas provides a good example. As noted at the beginning, 83% of Texas schools teach either no sex ed or abstinence-only education,[55] and yet Texas is first in the nation for repeat teen pregnancies,[56] fifth for teen pregnancies,[57] and third for HIV rates.[58] Clearly, if abstinence-only education was the best program, we would be doing better.

Texas is just one state, though, and we should look at the nation overall and see if the same trend holds true for all 50 states.

It does.

In a peer-reviewed 2011 paper by Drs. Stanger-Hall and Hall, they concluded that even after accounting for other factors, "The more strongly abstinence is emphasized in state laws and policies, the higher the average teenage pregnancy and birth rate."[59]

This doesn't mean it's wrong to emphasize abstinence—just that it **alone** is not enough to protect young people. Sooner or later young people **will** become sexually active, and in this case ignorance can be fatal, even to those who remained virgins until marriage.[60]

We are not saying that lack of comprehensive sex education is "the" only cause either. Clearly high teen pregnancy rates also correlate with socioeconomic status,[61] minority status,[62] and religiosity.[63] But these things are less easily addressed by changes in policy, whereas we **can** change what we teach in schools.

Nor are we saying that gains have not been made. In fact, teen pregnancy is at a historic low, and the rates have fallen in all 50 states,[64] largely due to improved contraceptive use.[65] It remains true, however, that states like Texas, New Mexico, Mississippi, Arkansas, Louisiana, Oklahoma, Kentucky and West Virginia are way behind everyone else and still lead the nation and the developed world in teen pregnancy rates.

Our main goal here has been to provide education on the various contraceptive and disease prevention options that are available, and we hope we have at least started that discussion between you and your partner. However, there are many additional topics that can be covered in a marital education class.

As one example, we did not cover the human reproductive system, but we are hoping the basics were covered in biology class. If not, www.innerbody.com provides basic terminology and explanations, as well as two-dimensional interactive diagrams and some three-dimensional diagrams that allow you to rotate and zoom on the various organs in the reproductive system. These are pretty cool and provide excellent anatomical education.

We also didn't cover sex, and if you are from a school wholly lacking sex ed, that could be a significant oversight. We recommend any of Dr. Ruth Westheimer's books, including *Sex for Dummies.*

Assuming you get past that hurdle, we didn't cover pregnancy, childbirth, or parenting either, and sooner or later these are life-changing issues that many couples will face.

Other important topics not covered here are consent and communication. Gone are the days when consent was not legally required after marriage. It is. Don't assume that you have consent just because you are married. Ask. Of course, that assumes you can communicate, and often that is problematic. How can one even get to using a condom for protection if one is too embarrassed to discuss the topic with a partner? Actually, how can a couple resolve **any** problems if they are not good communicators? Communication is vital to your relationship and to your health and safety.

However, such topics are beyond the scope of this little book, which seeks to leave you with only two messages:

1) Treble-up: use three forms of birth control.

2) Consider abstinence-plus–marital education and help reduce teen pregnancy and STI rates in your state.

Glossary

The following glossary is adapted from the one provided by Planned Parenthood at https://www.plannedparenthood.org/learn/glossary.

Abstinence: Not having sex with a partner. However, abstinence means different things to different people, and being abstinent won't protect you from all STIs if there is still some intimate contact or if an STI is contracted nonsexually.

Abstinence-only programs: Curricula that teach abstinence as the only morally correct option for unmarried people. They do not include information about the health benefits of condoms for the prevention of STIs and other methods of birth control for the prevention of unintended pregnancy.

Acquaintance rape: Sexual intercourse that is forced by someone the victim knows.

Acquired immune deficiency syndrome (AIDS): The most advanced stage of HIV disease.

Adolescence: That time of physical and emotional change that begins at puberty and ends at early adulthood.

Adrenarche: The time in early puberty when secondary sex characteristics begin to develop.

Age of consent: The age at which state law considers a person old enough to decide to have sex with a partner. Typically, age 16 or 18.

Age of majority: The age at which state law recognizes a person as a legal adult. Typically, age 18.

AIDS: See *acquired immune deficiency syndrome.*

Amenorrhea: A lack of menstruation.

Androgens: Certain hormones that stimulate male sexual development and secondary male sex characteristics. Large amounts are produced in men's testicles and small amounts are produced in women's ovaries. The most common androgen is testosterone.

Andropause: The gradual decline in sexual vigor due to decreasing levels of testosterone as men age. Similar to menopause in women.

Anesthesia: Medication that causes a loss of sensation and protects against pain during medical procedures.

Antibiotics: Medicines that are used to cure infections caused by bacteria, fungi, or protozoa.

Antibody: A protein developed by the immune system in response to a toxin introduced into the body.

Anus: The opening from the rectum from which solid waste (feces) leaves the body.

Areola: The dark area surrounding the nipples of women and men.

Atrophic vaginitis: A vaginal irritation without a discharge caused by the lower levels of estrogen that occur with increased age.

Backup birth control: Any method—including condoms, diaphragms, sponges, or withdrawal—that is used while waiting for another method to become effective or when another method fails. Some people also refer to emergency contraception as backup birth control.

Bacterial vaginosis (BV): Inflammation of the vulva and/or vagina—vaginitis—caused by a change in the balance of vaginal bacteria. BV isn't an STI, but having sex with a new partner, or multiple partners, may increase your risk for BV. Sex sometimes leads to BV if your partner's natural chemistry changes the balance in your vagina.

Balanitis: An inflammation of the glans and foreskin of the penis that can be caused by infections—including STIs—irritations, drugs, or other factors.

Barrier methods of birth control: Contraceptives that block sperm from entering the uterus. These are the male condom, female condom, diaphragm, cap, spermicide, and sponge.

Bartholin's glands: Two glands that provide lubrication during sexual excitement. They are located in the inner labia on each side of the opening to the vagina.

Basal body temperature method: A fertility awareness–based birth control method for predicting a woman's fertility by taking her temperature. Can be used for contraception or planning a pregnancy.

Birth canal: The passage from the uterus through the cervix and vagina through which a baby is pushed out of a woman's body during childbirth.

Birth control: Behaviors, devices, or medications used to avoid unintended pregnancy. Also, contraceptives.

Bladder: The organ that collects and stores urine produced by the kidney. The bladder is emptied through the urethra.

Blastocyst: The developing preembryo shortly before implantation when it is a hollow ball of cells.

Breasts: Two glands on the chests of women. Breasts are secondary sex characteristics in women. Like mammary glands in other mammals, they produce milk during and after pregnancy. Men also have breast tissue.

Bubo: A swollen gland and sore caused by chancroid.

Bulbourethral glands: The glands, also called "Cowper's glands," beneath the prostate gland and attached to the urethra. They produce an alkaline fluid—preejaculate or precum—that neutralizes the urethra in preparation for ejaculation. Preejaculate also reduces friction in the urethra, making it easier for semen to pass through.

BV: See *bacterial vaginosis.*

Calendar method: A method for predicting fertility in which women chart their menstrual cycles on a calendar. Can be used for contraception or to plan a pregnancy.

Candida: A type of yeast—*Candida albicans*—and a common cause of vaginitis. Yeast infections may also occur in the penis or scrotum. When they occur orally, they are called "thrush."

Cap: A firm, thimblelike rubber or silicone cup that is intended to fit securely on the cervix. Used with contraceptive jelly (spermicide), the cervical cap is a barrier method of birth control that is reversible and available only by prescription. The FemCap is the only cervical cap currently available in the U.S.

Celibacy: Not having sex.

Cervical cap: See *cap.*

Cervical mucus: The secretion from the lower end of the uterus into the vagina. It changes in quality and quantity throughout the menstrual cycle, especially around the time of ovulation.

Cervical mucus method: A fertility awareness–based method for predicting a woman's fertility by observing changes in cervical mucus. Can be used for contraception or for planning a pregnancy.

Cervicitis: An irritation of the cervix. May include abnormal discharge from the cervix that can look and feel like a vaginal discharge.

Cervix: The narrow, lower part—neck—of the uterus, with a narrow opening connecting the uterus to the vagina.

Cesarean section / C-section: Childbirth in which the baby is taken out of the uterus surgically.

Chancre: A sore on the skin or mucus membrane that is caused by syphilis during the first phase of infection.

Chancroid: A once common sexually transmitted bacterium that causes open genital sores, called "buboes." As few as 3 cases per year in the U.S.

Change of life: Common term for menopause.

***Chlamydia*:** A common, sexually transmitted bacterium that can cause sterility and arthritis in women and men. The disease it causes now bears its name—chlamydia.

Climax: An orgasm or to have an orgasm.

Clitoral hood: A small flap of skin formed by the inner labia that covers and protects the clitoris.

Clitoris: The female sex organ that is very sensitive to the touch. It is made of spongy tissue that swells with blood during sexual excitement. The external tip of the clitoris is located at the top of the vulva, where the inner lips meet. The inner structure of the clitoris includes a shaft and two crura (roots or legs) of tissue that extend up to five inches into a woman's body on both sides of her vagina to attach to the pubic bone. Networks of highly sensitive nerves extend from the crura in the pelvic area.

Cytomegalovirus (CMV): An infection that may be transmitted through sexual or intimate contact or at childbirth that may cause permanent disability, including hearing loss and mental retardation for infants and blindness and mental disorders for adults.

Coitus: Sex in which the penis enters the vagina. Also called "vaginal intercourse."

Colposcope: A viewing instrument with a bright light and magnifying lens that is used to examine the vagina and cervix. Colposcopes are not inserted into a woman's body.

Combination pill: A birth control pill that contains the hormones estrogen and progestin. Also, combined hormone contraceptives or combined oral contraceptives.

Comprehensive sex education: A medically accurate curriculum that provides young people with positive messages about sex and sexuality as natural, normal, healthy parts of life; includes information about abstinence as the best way to avoid STIs and unintended pregnancy; teaches that condoms reduce the risk of infection, including HIV, and that other forms of birth control also reduce the risk of unplanned pregnancy for young people who are sexually active; and provides opportunities to help young people develop relationship and communications skills to help them explore their own values, goals, and options as well as the values of their families and communities.

Conception: The moment when the preembryo attaches to the lining of the uterus and pregnancy begins. Sometimes used to describe the fertilization of the egg.

Condom: A sheath of thin rubber, plastic, or animal tissue that is worn on the penis during sexual intercourse. It is an over-the-counter, reversible barrier method of birth control, and it also reduces the risk of getting the most serious sexually transmitted infections.

Congenital syphilis: Syphilis that is transmitted from a woman to her fetus during pregnancy, leading to bone disorders, wasting, loss of sight and/or hearing, deformities, stillbirth, or death of the newborn.

Contraception/contraceptive: Any behavior, device, medication, or procedure used to prevent pregnancy.

Contraceptive creams and jellies: Substances containing spermicide, which block and immobilize sperm and prevent it from joining with the egg. These are over-the-counter reversible methods of birth control. Used with cervical caps, diaphragms and condoms.

Contraceptive film/c-film: A thin, two-inch square sheet of chemicals that is inserted deep into the vagina and melts into a thick liquid that blocks the entrance to the uterus with a spermicide. It immobilizes sperm and prevents it from joining with an egg. An over-the-counter reversible method of birth control. Most effective when used with a condom.

Contraceptive foam: A bubbling substance, inserted deep into the vagina, that blocks the entrance to the uterus with spermicide that immobilizes sperm, preventing it from joining with an egg. An over-the-counter reversible method of birth control. Most effective when used with a condom.

Contraceptive suppository: A solid capsule containing spermicide that, once inserted deep into the vagina, melts into a liquid to block and immobilize sperm, preventing it from joining with an egg. An over-the-counter reversible method of birth control. Most effective when used with a condom.

Copulation: Vaginal intercourse.

Corona: The edge of the glans of the penis.

Corpus cavernosa: Two strips of erectile tissue in the glans, shaft, and crura of the clitoris and along the sides of the penis that extend back into the pelvic floor. During sexual excitement, they fill with blood and become erect.

Corpus luteum: A mass of cells that form on an ovary and produces estrogens and progesterone following the release of an egg.

Corpus spongiosum: Erectile tissue that forms the glans of the clitoris and penis. In the penis, it runs from the glans along the underside of the shaft, surrounding the urethra.

Cowper's glands: The glands, also called "bulbourethral glands," beneath the prostate gland that are attached to the urethra. They produce a fluid—preejaculate or "precum"—that prepares the urethra for ejaculation. Preejaculate also reduces friction in the urethra, making it easier for semen to pass through.

Cremaster: The muscle that elevates the testicles as temperatures get colder or when the front or inner surface of the thigh is stimulated.

Cremaster reflex: The automatic response of the cremaster muscle, which elevates both testicles when exposed to cold. In response to thigh stimulation, only the testicle next to the stimulated thigh will be lifted.

Crura: Internal extensions of the corpus cavernosa of the clitoris and penis that attach to the pubic bone.

Cum: Slang for *ejaculate.*

Cystitis: An infection of the bladder. Also called "urinary tract infection" or "UTI."

CMV: See *cytomegalovirus.*

Dental dam: A stretchable square of latex used as a barrier during certain dental procedures. Also, sometimes used as a barrier for safer sex.

Depo-provera: The brand name of a progestin (depot medroxyprogesterone acetate [DMPA]) that is injected into the buttock or arm every 12 weeks to prevent pregnancy. It is a reversible method of birth control available only by prescription.

Depot medroxyprogesterone acetate (DMPA): Progestin found in Depo-Provera. Used for contraception.

Diabetic vulvitis: A yeast infection caused by contact with urine that has the high sugar content associated with diabetes.

Diaphragm: A soft rubber dome intended to fit securely over the cervix. Used with spermicide, the diaphragm is a reversible barrier method of birth control available only by prescription.

DMPA: See *depot medroxyprogesterone acetate.*

Douche: A spray of water or solution of medication into the vagina.

Dysmenorrhea: Pain or discomfort before or during menstruation.

Dyspareunia: Painful vaginal intercourse for women that may be caused by hormonal imbalances. Most likely to happen after menopause.

Egg: The reproductive cell in women; the largest cell in the human body.

Ejaculation: The moment when semen spurts out of the opening of the urethra in the glans of the penis.

Emergency contraception: Hormonal birth control pills used to prevent pregnancy after unprotected vaginal intercourse. Must be started within 120 hours (five days) of unprotected intercourse. The copper IUD can also be used as emergency contraception, if inserted within five days of unprotected intercourse to prevent pregnancy.

Endometriosis: The growth of endometrial tissue outside of the uterus, causing pain, especially before and during menstruation.

Endometrium: The lining of the uterus that develops every month in order to nourish a fertilized egg. The lining is shed during menstruation if there is no implantation of a fertilized egg.

Endorphin: A hormone that suppresses pain.

Epididymis: The tube leading from the testis to the vas deferens in which sperm are stored before ejaculation. It is tightly coiled on top of and behind the testis. The plural of *epididymis* is *epididymides.*

Epididymitis: An inflammation of the epididymis.

Erectile dysfunction: The inability to become erect or maintain an erection with a partner.

Erectile tissue: Spongy tissue in the body that stiffens when filled with blood. See *vasocongestion.*

Erection: A "hard" penis when it becomes full of blood and stiffens. See *vasocongestion.*

Estrogen: A hormone commonly made in a woman's ovaries. Estrogen's major feminizing effects are seen during puberty, menstruation, and pregnancy.

Estrus: The cyclic period of fertility and sexual receptivity in subprimate female animals (vertebrates).

External sex and reproductive organs: The sex organs and structures on the outside of the body that are primarily used during sexual activity. These include the vulva in a woman and the penis and scrotum in a man.

Failure rate: The number of women who become pregnant each year out of every 100 who use a birth control method.

Fallopian tube: One of two narrow tubes that carry the egg from the ovary to the uterus.

Family planning: Voluntary planning and action by individuals to have the number of children they want, when they want them.

FAMs: See *fertility awareness–based methods.*

Fecundity: Technically, the physical ability of a woman or couple to have a child. Often used as a synonym for *fertility.*

Female condom: A polyurethane pouch with flexible rings at each end that is inserted deep into the vagina like a diaphragm. It is an over-the-counter reversible barrier method of birth control that provides protection against many sexually transmitted infections. Formerly called "a vaginal pouch." May also be used rectally.

Female ejaculation: The spurting of fluid out of the urethra during intense sexual excitement or orgasm. The fluid is most likely secreted by the Skene's glands, which are located in the vulva near the opening of the urethra. Female ejaculation may be associated with stimulation of the G-spot and occurs in 1 out of 10 women.

Female prostate glands: Term used by some to describe the Skene's glands in a woman's vulva, which may secrete a fluid similar to the fluid produced by the prostate gland in men.

FemCap: See *cap.*

Fertility: The ability of women or couples to have children. Technically, the childbearing performance of individuals, couples, groups, or populations (i.e., the number of births they have).

Fertility awareness–based methods (FAMs): Ways to prevent or plan pregnancy by predicting ovulation based on understanding a woman's fertility cycle.

Fertility cycle: Also called the menstrual cycle. The monthly recurrence of ovulation, the shedding of the lining of the uterus, and the body's preparation for another ovulation.

Fertility rate: The number of live births per 1,000 women of reproductive age (15–44).

Fertilization: The joining of an egg and sperm that forms the zygote.

Fetus: The organism that develops from the embryo at the end of about eight weeks of pregnancy (10 weeks after a woman's last menstrual period) and receives nourishment through the placenta.

Fidelity: Strict observance of promises, especially of sexual faithfulness.

Follicle: A cavity and sac in the ovary that contains a maturing egg.

Follicle-stimulating hormone (FSH): Made by the pituitary gland, it stimulates the growth of the egg in women and the development of sperm in men.

Fordyce spots: Small, slightly bumpy yellowish or white papules or spots on the inside of the cheeks or lips, or on the glans or shaft of the penis, or the labia of the vulva. They are sebaceous glands and 50 to 100 may appear in one area. They are completely harmless, are not sexually transmitted, and are not infectious.

Foreskin: A retractable tube of skin that covers and protects the glans (head) of the penis.

Frenulum: In women, the highly sensitive tissue where the inner labia join below the glans of the clitoris. In men, the highly sensitive, triangular piece of skin just below the glans of the penis.

FSH: See *Follicle-stimulating hormone.*

Gamete: A reproductive cell—egg or sperm.

Genital herpes: An infection of herpes simplex virus types 1 or 2 in the area of the anus, buttocks, cervix, penis, vagina, or vulva. Very often there are no symptoms, while the most common symptom is a cluster of blistery sores.

Genitals: External sex and reproductive organs: the vulva in women, the penis and scrotum in men. Sometimes, the internal reproductive organs are also called genitals.

Genital warts: Soft, flesh-colored growths caused by several types of the human papillomavirus. They may look like miniature cauliflower florets and are usually painless, but may itch.

Glans: The soft, highly sensitive tip of the clitoris or penis. In men, the opening to the urethra is located in the glans. Also called the "head" of the penis.

Gonadotropins: Hormones secreted by the pituitary gland that trigger puberty by stimulating the ovaries of women and the testes of men.

Gonads: The organs that produce reproductive cells—the ovaries of women, the testes of men.

Gonorrhea: A sexually transmitted bacterium that can cause sterility, arthritis, and heart problems.

Gräfenberg spot (G-spot): An area of tissue, located about one-third of the way along the upper wall of the vagina. Stimulation of the G-spot leads to intense sexual arousal and orgasm in some women and is also associated with female ejaculation.

Gynecologist: A medical doctor who specializes in women's sexual and reproductive health.

Gynecology: Sexual and reproductive health care for women.

Gynecomastia: A usually temporary condition during puberty in which the breasts of boys become larger and appear more feminine.

HBV: See *Hepatitis B virus.*

Herpes simplex virus (HSV): An infection of herpes simplex virus types 1 or 2 in the area of the anus, buttocks, cervix, mouth, penis, vagina, or vulva. Very often there are no symptoms, while the most common symptom is a cluster of blistery sores.

HIV: See *Human immunodeficiency virus.*

Honeymoon cystitis: A bladder infection (urinary tract infection or "UTI") in a woman that is caused by frequent vaginal intercourse—for example, during a honeymoon. Clean hands and nails, as well as urination after sex, may help to prevent a UTI.

Hormonal contraceptives: Prescription methods of birth control that use hormones to prevent pregnancy. These include the implant, the Mirena IUD, the patch, the pill, the ring, and the shot.

Hormones: Chemicals that cause changes in our bodies and influence how glands and organs work.

HPV: See *Human papillomavirus.*

HSV: See *Herpes simplex virus.*

Human immunodeficiency virus (HIV): An infection that weakens the body's ability to fight disease and can cause AIDS.

Human papillomavirus (HPV): Any of more than 100 different types of virus, some of which may cause genital warts. Others may cause cancer of the anus, cervix, penis, throat, or vulva.

Hydrocele: An accumulation of fluid in a testicle.

Hymen: The thin fleshy tissue that stretches across part of the opening to the vagina in some, but not all, girls.

Implanon: The brand name of a contraceptive implant.

Implant: A thin, flexible plastic implant about the size of a cardboard matchstick. It is inserted under the skin of the upper arm. It releases a progestin that prevents ovulation and fertilization. Can be used for up to three to five years to prevent pregnancy. The implant is a reversible hormonal method of birth control available only by prescription. Implanon and Nexplanon are brand names of implants.

Implantation: The attachment of the preembryo to the lining of the uterus, which begins about six days after fertilization and is complete in three to four days. Marks the beginning of pregnancy.

Impotence: The inability to have an erection. *Erectile dysfunction* is now the preferred term.

Inner lips: The labia of the vulva that surround the clitoris and the openings to the urethra and vagina. Also called "labia minora."

Intercourse: Sexual activity in which the penis is inserted into the vagina (vaginal intercourse) or the rectum (anal intercourse).

Internal sex and reproductive organs: The organs inside the body that are responsible for producing, moving, and nourishing human reproductive cells. Internal reproductive organs that are sensitive or respond to sexual stimulation are also called "sex organs."

Intrauterine device (IUD): A small device made of plastic, which may contain copper or a hormone, that is inserted into the uterus by a health care provider to prevent pregnancy. A reversible method of birth control, available only by prescription.

Intrauterine system (IUS): A small IUD made of plastic that contains the hormone progestin and is inserted into the uterus by a health care provider to prevent pregnancy. A reversible method of birth control available only by prescription. The brand name of the IUS is Mirena.

Introitus: The tissue of the inner vulva that frames the opening to the vagina.

IUD: See *intrauterine device.*

IUS: See *intrauterine system.*

Jock itch: A very common fungal skin infection in the genital area of men that is caused by wearing tight clothing, sweating, or not drying the genitals carefully after bathing. It can cause a reddish, scaly rash that can become inflamed, very itchy, and painful.

Labia majora: The outer lips of the vulva.

Labia minora: The inner lips of the vulva.

Lactational amenorrhea method (LAM): Breastfeeding as birth control for up to six months after childbirth.

Lactobacilli: Bacteria present in healthy vaginas of women. They help prevent vaginitis by limiting the growth of *Candida*—a yeast.

LAM: See *lactational amenorrhea method.*

Laparoscope: A rodlike instrument with a light and viewing lens. Often used for tubal sterilization procedures.

Laparoscopy: A very common method of visualizing the interior of the abdomen with a laparoscope. Used in tubal sterilization. It involves injection of a harmless gas to help see the reproductive organs through a small incision near the navel, which allows the positioning of a laparoscope and use of an instrument to block the fallopian tubes.

Laparotomy: A type of major surgery, requiring a two- to five-inch abdominal incision through which, in tubal sterilization, the fallopian tubes are located and blocked.

Leukorrhea: A white, yellow, or greenish, sticky vaginal discharge that is normal during adolescence, pregnancy, and other times when a woman's hormone levels are changing.

Levonorgestrel: A synthetic progestin, similar to the hormone progesterone, which is produced by the body to regulate the menstrual cycle. Used in certain birth control pills, the Mirena IUD, and Plan B emergency contraceptives.

LGV: See *Lymphogranuloma venereum.*

Lobes: Groups of alveoli sacs in women's breasts.

Lubricant: In women, the slippery liquid that is secreted from the walls of the vagina and the Bartholin's glands during sexual arousal in order to facilitate vaginal intercourse. In men, the slippery liquid secreted by the Cowper's glands in order to facilitate ejaculation and sperm motility. Also, an oil-based, water-based, or silicone-based product used to decrease friction during sex.

Luteinizing hormone (LH): One type of gonadatropin, a hormone secreted by the pituitary gland. Triggers ovulation in women and the production of testosterone in men. There are over-the-counter test kits for detecting LH. Also known as lutropin.

Lymphocele: A small swelling caused by the collection of lymphatic fluid. May occur on the penis.

Lymphogranuloma venereum (LGV): A form of chlamydia, most common in tropical regions. Increasingly found in the U.S.

Mammary glands: Organs in a woman's breasts that produce milk.

Mammogram: X-ray photographs of the breasts that can detect cancerous tumors before they can be felt.

Menarche: The time of a girl's first menstruation.

Menopause: The time at midlife when menstruation stops; a woman's last period; usually occurs between the age of 45 and 55. "Surgical menopause," however, results from removal of the ovaries, and may occur earlier.

Menorrhagia: Menstrual bleeding that is heavier or longer lasting than usual.

Menses: The discharge during menstruation.

Menstrual cup: A latex or silicone receptacle that fits over the cervix to collect menstrual flow.

Menstrual cycle: The time from the first day of one period to the first day of the next period. In women of reproductive age, about age 15–44, it is the period in which the lining of the uterus is shed whenever implantation does not happen, followed by the regrowth of the lining of the uterus in preparation for implantation.

Menstrual flow: Blood, fluid, and tissue that are passed out of the uterus during the beginning of the menstrual cycle. Often called a "period."

Menstrual synchrony: Women having their periods at the same time because they live closely together.

Menstrual suppression: The use of hormonal treatments—usually birth control pills—to prevent periods.

Menstruation: The flow of blood, fluid, and tissue out of the uterus and through the vagina that usually lasts from three to seven days.

Milk ducts: The passages in women's breasts through which milk flows from the alveoli to the nipple.

Mini-laparotomy: A very common surgical approach used in tubal sterilization that involves making a small incision on the lower abdomen through which the fallopian tubes can be located and blocked.

Mini-pills: Birth control pills that contain only the hormone progestin. More correctly called "progestin-only pills."

Miscarriage: The loss of a pregnancy before 20 weeks' gestation—before the embryo or fetus can live outside the uterus.

Molluscum contagiosum: A virus that can be sexually transmitted, causing small, pinkish-white, waxy, round, polyp-like growths in the genital area or on the thighs.

Monogamy: A relationship in which both people date or have sex only with one another and no one else.

Mons veneris: The fleshy, triangular mound above the vulva that is covered with pubic hair in adult women. It cushions the pubic bone.

Morning-after pills: Emergency hormonal contraception that is started within 120 hours (five days) of unprotected vaginal intercourse to decrease the risk of unintended pregnancy.

Mucus method: A fertility awareness–based method for predicting a woman's fertility by observing changes in her cervical mucus. Can be used for contraception or for planning a pregnancy.

Müllerian ducts: Two structures in the embryo that develop into the female reproductive tract.

Multiparous: Having given birth more than once.

Natural family planning: Fertility awareness–based methods of contraception. Inaccurately suggests that other methods are unnatural, which is why the term *fertility-awareness method* is preferred.

Nexplanon: A brand name for an implant. The Nexplanon implant is radiopaque, meaning that it can be tracked by X-ray or other imaging methods.

NGU: See *Nongonococcal urethritis.*

Nidation: Implantation, the attachment of the preembryo to the lining of the uterus, which begins about six days after fertilization and is complete in three to four days. The beginning of pregnancy.

Nipple: The dark tissue in the center of the areola of each breast in women and men that can stand erect when stimulated by touch or cold. In a woman's breast, the nipple may release milk that is produced by the breast.

Nocturnal emission: A wet dream; sexual arousal and ejaculation while sleeping, which most often occurs among young men during adolescence or older men who are sexually abstinent.

Nocturnal orgasm: A sexual climax during sleep.

Nocturnal penile tumescence (NPT): Spontaneous erection during sleep that occurs among healthy men from birth through old age. NPT usually occurs about two or three times a night, lasting for a total of two or three hours.

Nongonococcal urethritis (NGU): An inflammation of the urethra that is not caused by gonorrhea—often caused by chlamydia.

Nonoxynol-9: A chemical that immobilizes sperm that is used in most spermicides in the U.S.

Nonparous: Having never given birth.

Norgestrel: A kind of progestin used in some hormonal contraceptives.

NPT: See *nocturnal penile tumescence.*

Nulliparous: Having never given birth.

Nuptial: Regarding marriage.

NuvaRing: The brand name of a ring that contains hormones and is inserted in the vagina to prevent pregnancy. NuvaRing is a reversible hormonal method of birth control available only by prescription. Also called "the ring."

Oocyte: An immature ovum, egg.

Oophorectomy: Surgical removal of an ovary.

Oral contraceptive: The birth control pill.

Oral herpes: An infection of the mouth with herpes simplex virus 1 or herpes simplex virus 2.

Orchiectomy: The surgical removal of one or both testicles. Usually performed to treat cancer or for genital reconstruction surgery.

Orchitis: Inflammation of a testicle.

Ortho Evra: Ortho Evra, a transdermal contraceptive patch, is a reversible hormonal method of birth control available only by prescription. Also called "the patch."

Outer lips: See *labia majora.*

Ovarian cyst: A growth on an ovary, usually small, fluid-filled, and not cancerous. May cause abdominal pain or irregular periods. Most often resolves on its own.

Ovaries: The two organs that store eggs in a woman's body. Ovaries also produce hormones, including estrogen, progesterone, and testosterone.

Over-the-counter: Available without a prescription.

Oviduct: Fallopian tube, one of two narrow tubes that carry the egg from the ovary to the uterus.

Ovulation: The time when an ovary releases an egg.

Pap test: A procedure used to examine the cells of the cervix in order to detect abnormal, precancerous, or cancerous growths. It is also called a "Pap smear."

ParaGard/Copper T 380A: An IUD that contains copper and can be left in place for up to 12 years.

Parous: Having given birth.

Parthenogenesis: The development of an unfertilized egg into an organism. Common in some animals, but is not yet known to occur in humans, although childbearing women have claimed to be virgins. Human eggs can be convinced to start reproducing without being fertilized, but scientists doubt such cells would ever produce a child. If it did, the child would be female due to lack of a Y chromosome. If parthogenesis were possible, it would mean that abstinence has a higher failure rate than is usually attributed to it.

Parturition: Childbirth.

Pearly pink papules/pearly penile papules: Tiny bumps that ring the edge of the head of the penis in 1 out of 3 men. Flesh-colored or a little lighter, they are shaped like smooth little domes. Although they may be sensitive to touch, they are not harmful and are not sexually transmitted. They can be removed with laser treatment.

Pediculosis: An infestation of pubic lice: pediculus pubis. Also known as "crabs."

Pelvic exam: A physical examination of the vulva, vagina, cervix, uterus, and ovaries that usually includes taking cervical cells for a Pap test and a manual exam of the internal pelvic organs.

Pelvic girdle: The bony and muscular structure inside a woman's body that supports her internal sex and reproductive organs.

Pelvic inflammatory disease (PID): An infection of a woman's internal reproductive system that can lead to sterility, ectopic pregnancy, and chronic pain. It is often caused by sexually transmitted infections, such as gonorrhea and chlamydia.

Pelvic tuberculosis: A rare, chronic bacterial infection of a woman's reproductive organs. Can cause infertility.

Penis: A man's reproductive and sex organ that is formed of three columns of spongy tissue—two corpora cavernosa and the corpus spongiosum. The spongy tissue fills with blood during sexual excitement, a process known as erection. Urine and seminal fluid pass through the penis.

Perimenopause: The period of change leading to menopause.

Perineum: The area between the anus and the vulva or scrotum.

Period: See *Menstruation.*

Periodic abstinence: Not having vaginal intercourse during the "unsafe days" of a woman's fertile phase in order to prevent pregnancy.

Pessary: A device inserted into the vagina to treat a prolapsed uterus. Older types of pessaries were used as barrier birth control methods.

Pheromones: Odors given off by animals, including humans, to attract others sexually.

Phimosis: A condition in which the foreskin of the penis is too tight to be pulled back.

PID: See *pelvic inflammatory disease.*

Pill, the: A common expression for oral hormonal contraception.

Pituitary gland: Located under the brain, the organ that produces hormones that regulate growth, reproduction, and sexual activity.

Placenta: The organ formed on the wall of the uterus by the developing embryo that provides oxygen and other nourishment from the woman to the fetus and through which waste products are eliminated from the fetus.

Plan B: The brand name for oral hormonal emergency contraception, the morning-after pill.

PMS: See *premenstrual syndrome.*

Polycystic ovary syndrome: Various symptoms that result from small benign growths on the ovaries, including lack of menstruation, excessive body hair, and infertility.

Polyps: Small benign growths (tumors) common in the uterus and on the cervix or throat.

Postexposure prophylaxis: Medication provided immediately after possible exposure to a sexually transmitted infection, including HIV, which is intended to prevent infection.

Postpartum: The first few weeks after childbirth.

Postpartum depression: Depression in a woman following childbirth.

Preejaculate ("precum"): The liquid, which is produced by Cowper's glands, that oozes out of the penis during sexual excitement before ejaculation. Does not contain sperm, but may pick up sperm remaining in the urethra from previous ejaculations.

Pregnancy: A condition in which a woman carries a developing offspring in her uterus. It begins with the implantation of the preembryo and progresses through the embryonic and fetal stages until birth. It lasts about nine months from implantation to birth. If clinically measured from a woman's last menstrual period, it lasts 10 months.

Premenstrual syndrome (PMS): Emotional and physical symptoms that appear a few days before and during menstruation, including depression, fatigue, feeling bloated, and irritability.

Prepuce: Foreskin.

Preputial glands: The organs that secrete a fluid that combines with bacteria and body oils to form smegma. Several are located under the foreskin and clitoral hood. Others are located under the corona of the glans of the penis and on either side of the frenulum. Also called Tyson's glands.

Priapism: A prolonged and painful erection of the penis without sexual stimulation that is caused by too much blood flow into the corpus cavernosa.

Primary sex characteristics: Body organs and reproductive structures and functions, which differ between women and men. The differences include the external and internal sex and reproductive organs. It also includes a woman's ability to produce eggs and a man's ability to produce sperm.

Primary syphilis: The first stage of infection during which an open sore called a chancre develops.

Progesterone: A hormone produced in the ovaries of women that is important in the regulation of puberty, menstruation, and pregnancy.

Progestin: A synthetic progesterone.

Prophylactic: A device or treatment used to prevent infection; also the condom.

Prostaglandins: Hormones that are used to induce uterine contractions for childbirth.

Prostate: A gland the size of a golf ball that is located below the bladder in men and produces a fluid that helps sperm move. Very sensitive to the touch.

Prostatitis: An enlargement and inflammation of the prostate gland that results in a dull persistent pain in the lower back, glans of the penis, scrotum, and testes. There may also be a thin mucus discharge from the penis, especially in the morning.

Puberty: The time between childhood and adulthood when girls and boys mature physically and sexually. Puberty is marked by changes such as breast development and menstruation in girls and facial hair growth and ejaculation in boys.

Pubic hair: Hair that grows around the sex organs of women and men. Pubic hair is a secondary sex characteristic that appears during puberty.

Pubic lice: Tiny insects that can be sexually transmitted. They live in pubic hair and cause intense itching in the genitals or anus.

Rectum: The lowest end of the intestine before the anus, where solid waste (feces) is stored.

Refractory period: The time after ejaculation during which a man is not able to have an erection.

Reproductive cell: A unique cell—egg in women, sperm in men—that can join with its opposite to make reproduction possible.

Reproductive organs: In women: the fallopian tubes, ovaries, uterus, and vagina. In men: the penis, prostate, and testes.

Rhythm method: Outdated name for what is now called the calendar method of fertility awareness.

Rugae: The folds of tissue in the walls of the vagina.

Scabies: Tiny mites that can be sexually transmitted. They burrow under the skin, causing intense itching, usually at night, and small bumps or rashes that appear in small curling lines. They are especially found on the penis; between the fingers; on buttocks, breasts, wrists, and thighs; and around the navel.

Scrotum: A sac of skin, divided into two parts, enclosing the testes, epididymides, and parts of the vasa deferentia.

Secondary sex characteristics: Features of the body that are caused by hormones, develop during puberty, and last through adult life. For women, these include breast development and widened hips. For men, they include facial hair development. Both men and women develop pubic hair and underarm hair.

Secondary syphilis: The second stage of the infection, during which a rash and fever develop.

Semen: Fluid containing sperm that is ejaculated during sexual excitement. Semen is composed of fluid from the seminal vesicles, fluid from the prostate, and sperm from the testes.

Seminal fluid: A fluid that nourishes and helps sperm to move. Made in the seminal vesicles.

Seminal vesicle: One of two small organs located beneath the bladder and connected to the urethra that produce seminal fluid.

Seminiferous tubules: A network of tiny tubules in the testes that constantly produce sperm. Seminiferous tubules also produce androgens, the sex hormones associated with masculinization.

Sex cell: A reproductive cell. See *gamete*.

Sexually transmitted disease (STD): A sexually transmitted infection that has produced symptoms. Often used interchangeably with *sexually transmitted infection.*

Sexually transmitted infection (STI): An STD that may have or may not (yet) have caused disease symptoms.

Skene's glands. Two glands that produce fluid during female ejaculation. They are located on opposite sides of the opening to a woman's urethra. Also called "paraurethral glands" or "female prostate glands."

Smegma: A sticky, white, unpleasant-smelling substance produced under the foreskin at the glans of the penis and clitoris. It is formed by secretions from the Tyson's glands, bacteria, and body oils.

Somatotropin: The human growth hormone secreted by the pituitary gland.

Sperm: The reproductive cells in men, produced in the seminiferous tubules of the testes.

Spermarche: The time when sperm is first produced by the testes of a boy.

Spermatogenesis: The process of producing sperm. Occurs in the seminiferous tubules of the testes.

Spermicides: Chemicals used to immobilize and kill sperm.

Spirochete: The organism that causes syphilis.

Spotting: Usually, light bleeding between menstrual periods, which may only be seen on toilet tissue after wiping. Normal spotting is associated, for example, with ovulation, the use of some hormonal methods of birth control, the onset of menstruation, and perimenopause. Though not always abnormal, spotting during pregnancy or after vaginal intercourse should be discussed with one's health care provider. It can be a sign of endometriosis, uterine fibroids, vaginal adhesions or polyps, or cancer.

Standard Days Method: A fertility awareness-based method for predicting a woman's fertility by tracking her cycle on a string of CycleBeads. Can be used for contraception by women whose cycles are no shorter than 26 days or longer than 32 days.

STD: See *sexually transmitted disease.*

Sterilization: Surgical methods of birth control intended to be permanent—blocking of the fallopian tubes for women or the vas deferens for men.

STI: See *sexually transmitted infection.*

Syphilis: A sexually transmitted infection that can lead to disfigurement, neurological disorders, and death.

Temperature method: A fertility awareness-based method for predicting fertility in which women chart when ovulation occurs by taking their temperature every morning before getting out of bed. Can be used for contraception or for planning pregnancy.

Tertiary syphilis: The third phase of the infection during which multiple organ damage and failures occur.

Testes: Two ball-like glands inside the scrotum that produce hormones, including testosterone. Each testis also encloses several hundred small lobes, which contain the tiny, threadlike seminiferous tubules that produce sperm. Also called "testicles," the testes are sensitive to the touch.

Testicles: See *testes.*

Testosterone: An androgen that is produced in the testes of men and in smaller amounts in the ovaries of women.

Thelarche: The time when a girl's breasts begin to develop.

Triphasic combination pill: An oral contraceptive with varying doses of estrogen and progestin during a 28-day cycle.

Tubal ligation: Surgical blocking of the fallopian tubes by tying them off. A form of tubal sterilization.

Tubal sterilization: Blocking of the fallopian tubes by any of a variety of methods.

Tubectomy: The surgical removal of a fallopian tube.

Tumescence: Erection and enlargement of the sex organs, especially the clitoris and penis, during sexual arousal.

Two-day method: A fertility awareness-based method of contraception in which a woman observes whether or not she has had cervical mucus two days in a row.

Tyson's glands: The organs that secrete a fluid that combines with bacteria and body oils to form smegma. Several are located under the foreskin and clitoral hood. Others are located under the corona of the glans of the penis and on either side of the frenulum. Also called preputial glands.

Ureters: The two tubes that lead from the kidneys to the bladder.

Urethra: The tube from which women and men urinate. The urethra empties the bladder and carries urine to the urethral opening. In men, the urethra runs through the penis and also carries ejaculate and preejaculate during sexual activities and nocturnal emission.

Urinary tract infection (UTI): A bacterial infection of the bladder (also called "cystitis"), the ureters, or the urethra.

Uterus: The pear-shaped, muscular reproductive organ from which women menstruate and the womb where normal pregnancy develops.

UTI: See *urinary tract infection.*

Vagina: The stretchable passage that connects a woman's outer sex organs, the vulva, with the cervix and uterus. The vagina has three functions: to allow menstrual flow to leave the body, to allow sexual penetration to occur and to allow a fetus to pass through during vaginal delivery.

Vaginal atrophy: Thinning and irritation of the folds of the walls of the vagina caused by the normal reduction in the secretion of estrogen during perimenopause and after menopause.

Vaginal contraceptive film (VCF): A thin, two-inch square sheet of chemicals that is inserted deep into the vagina and melts into a thick liquid that blocks the entrance to the uterus with a spermicide. It immobilizes sperm and prevents it from joining with an egg. An over-the-counter, reversible barrier method of birth control. Most effective when used with a condom.

Vaginal intercourse: Sex in which a penis enters a vagina.

Vaginal lubrication: During sexual arousal, the secretion of a slippery fluid from the blood vessels that "perspires" through the rugae of the walls of the vagina into the vaginal canal to facilitate penetration.

Vaginitis: An irritation of the vagina or vulva.

Values: Ideas about what is right, worthwhile, or moral.

Varicocele: An enlargement of one or more of the veins that carry blood away from the testis. It can reduce blood flow and increase the temperature of the testicle, thereby causing infertility. Similar to varicose veins that occur in the leg.

Vas deferens: A long, narrow tube that carries sperm from each epididymis to the seminal vesicles during ejaculation. The plural of *vas deferens* is *vasa deferentia.*

Vasectomy: Surgical blocking of the vasa deferentia in men that is intended to provide permanent birth control.

Vasocongestion: An increase in the amount of blood in certain body tissues (breasts, clitoris, inner labia, nipples, penis) that is caused by sexual arousal. Also causes sex flushes (blushing of the skin) and lubrication of the vagina.

VD: Venereal disease (outdated). See *sexually transmitted disease.*

Viability: The ability of a fetus to survive outside a woman's body.

Virginity: The status of never having had sexual intercourse. People may have different definitions of virginity.

Vulva: A woman's external sex organs, including the clitoris, labia (majora and minora), opening to the vagina (introitus), opening to the urethra, and two Bartholin's glands.

Wet dreams: Erotic imaging during sleep that causes ejaculation in men and lubrication in women. See *nocturnal emission.*

Withdrawal: Pulling the penis out of the vagina before ejaculation in order to avoid pregnancy. A reversible, behavioral method of birth control.

X chromosome: The sex-differentiating chromosome that occurs twice in females and once in males.

Y chromosome: The sex-differentiating chromosome that occurs once in males and does not occur in females.

Yeast infection: Usually, a type of vaginitis caused by an overgrowth of the yeast *Candida albicans.* Yeast infections may also occur in the penis or scrotum. When they occur orally, they are referred to as "thrush."

Zika: A virus that's spread through mosquito bites and through the semen of an infected person. Most people who get Zika have no symptoms or ones that are very mild. In pregnancy, Zika can cause serious problems, including miscarriage and babies being born with brain and eye problems, smaller than normal heads, and developmental problems.

Zygote: The single-celled organism that results from the joining of the egg and sperm.

Notes

---

1 Kearney M. S. & Levine P. B., Why is the teen birth rate in the United States so high and why does it matter? J. Econ. Perspect. 26(2):141–66 (2012). Abstract available online at https://www.ncbi.nlm.nih.gov/pubmed/22792555. (Kearney and Levine write: "Teens in the United States are far more likely to give birth than in any other industrialized country in the world. U.S. teens are two and a half times as likely to give birth as compared to teens in Canada, around four times as likely as teens in Germany or Norway, and almost 10 times as likely as teens in Switzerland. Among more developed countries, Russia has the next highest teen birth rate after the United States, but an American teenage girl is still around 25 percent more likely to give birth than her counterpart in Russia.")

2 Power to Decide [formerly the National Campaign to Prevent Teen and Unplanned Pregnancy], Teen pregnancy rate comparison, 2013. Available online at https://powertodecide.org/what-we-do/information/national-state-data/teen-pregnancy-rate. According to more recent 2020 data at https://worldpopulationreview.com/states/teen-pregnancy-rates-by-state/, Texas is now tied with New Mexico for seventh highest teen pregnancy rate.

3 Teen Pregnancy Rate by State 2020, available online at https://worldpopulationreview.com/states/teen-pregnancy-rates-by-state/ ("Texas has the highest rate of repeat-teen births.")

4 Texas Freedom Network, Conspiracy of silence: Sexuality education in Texas public schools in 2015–2016. Available in 2017 online at https://tfn.org/new-tfn-education-fund-study-texas-is-failing-on-sex-education/, now available from Author.

5 Excerpted from Henry J. Kaiser Family Foundation, Sexual health of adolescents and young adults in the United States (2014). Available online at http://kff.org/womens-health-policy/fact-sheet/sexual-health-of-adolescents-and-young-adults-in-the-united-states/.

6 *Id.*, based on data from the CDC.

7 Guttmacher Institute, State facts about unintended pregnancy: Texas. Available online at https://www.guttmacher.org/sites/default/files/factsheet/tx_18.pdf.

8 Thomson-DeVeaux A., How defunding Planned Parenthood could affect health care, FiveThirtyEight (2017). Available online at https://fivethirtyeight.com/features/how-defunding-planned-parenthood-could-affect-health-care/. (Thomson-DeVeaux wrote: "Texas . . . embarked on a series of efforts to divert funding away from Planned Parenthood in 2011. First, the legislature instituted broad cuts to family planning services, spurring the closure of 82 clinics, one-third of which were affiliated with Planned Parenthood.") For more information on Texas efforts to defund reproductive health care, see Department of Health Policy, School of Public Health and Health Services, George Washington University, *Deteriorating Access to Women's Health Services in Texas: Potential Effects of the Women's Health Program Affiliate Rule* (2012). Available online at http://s3.amazonaws.com/static.texastribune.org/media/documents/GWU_WHP_study.pdf. See also Lee J., Charts: This is what happens when you defund Planned Parenthood, MotherJones (2013). Available online at http://www.motherjones.com/politics/2013/03/what-happens-when-you-defund-planned-parenthood.

9 Stevenson A. J., et al., Effect of removal of Planned Parenthood from the Texas Women's Health Program, N. Engl. J. Med. 374:853–860 (2016). Available online at http://www.nejm.org/doi/full/10.1056/NEJMsa1511902. (Stevenson et al. wrote: "The percentage of women who underwent childbirth covered by Medicaid within 18 months increased from 7.0% to 8.4% in the

counties with [now closed] Planned Parenthood affiliates and decreased from 6.4% to 5.9% in the counties without Planned Parenthood affiliates [estimated difference in differences, 1.9 percentage points; P = 0.01].")

[10] Hoffman S. D. & Maynard R. A. (eds.), *Kids Having Kids: Economic Costs and Social Consequences of Teen Pregnancy* (2nd ed.) (Washington, DC: Urban Institute Press, 2008), cited in U.S. Department of Health and Human Services, Teen pregnancy and childbearing (2019). Available online at https://www.hhs.gov/ash/oah/adolescent-development/reproductive-health-and-teen-pregnancy/teen-pregnancy-and-childbearing/index.html.

[11] Selby W. G., Democratic legislators say more than half of Texas births funded by Medicaid, PolitiFact Texas (2012). Available online at http://www.politifact.com/texas/statements/2012/mar/24/elliott-naishtat/democratic-legislators-say-more-half-texas-births-/. (Selby wrote: "[Texas Health and Human Services Commission] spokesman Geoffrey Wool . . . add[ed] that in 2010, 56.9 percent of Texas births—or 220,899 out of 388,447 total births—were covered by Medicaid, at an average cost of $11,600.")

[12] Guttmacher Institute, State facts about unintended pregnancy. Available online at https://www.guttmacher.org/fact-sheet/state-facts-about-unintended-pregnancy-texas#7. (Guttmacher reported that in 2010 "Texas spent the most ($2.9 billion)" in public funds on unintended pregnancies)

[13] Shuger L., *Teen Pregnancy and High School Dropout: What Communities Can Do to Address These Issues* (Washington, DC: The National Campaign to Prevent Teen and Unplanned Pregnancy and America's Promise Alliance, 2012), available online at https://powertodecide.org/what-we-do/information/resource-library/teen-pregnancy-and-high-school-dropout. (Shuger wrote that "fully 30 percent of teen girls who have dropped out of high school cite pregnancy or parenthood as a key reason. . . . According to the Alliance for Excellent Education [*The High Cost of High School Dropouts: What the Nation Pays for Inadequate High Schools* (2008)], it is estimated that over the course of his or her lifetime, a single high school dropout costs the nation approximately $260,000 in lost earnings, taxes, and productivity. Put another way, if students who dropped out of the Class of 2011 had graduated from high school, the nation's economy would likely benefit from nearly $154 billion in additional income over the course of their lifetimes.")

[14] HIV is human immunodeficiency virus, which will eventually cause AIDS—acquired immunodeficiency syndrome—and death if left untreated.

[15] CDC, *Texas—2015 State Health Profile* (n.d.). Available online at https://www.cdc.gov/nchhstp/stateprofiles/pdf/texas_profile.pdf.

[16] Corlis N., Ten U.S. Cities with Most Positive STD [Sexually Transmitted Disease] Tests (2015). Available online at https://www.stdcheck.com/blog/top-10-us-cities-positive-std-tests/. *Cf.* Different surveys include different diseases, and thus STD statistics are highly variable. This particular survey did not include herpes simplex virus 1 (HSV1) or hepatitis A, but did include chlamydia, gonorrhea, HSV-2, hepatitis B and C, HIV-1 and -2, and syphilis.

[17] American Sexual Health Association, Statistics (2020). Available online at http://www.ashasexualhealth.org/stdsstis/statistics/. (The American Sexual Health Association writes that the CDC "estimates that nearly 20 million new STIs occur every year [in the United States], half of those among young people aged 15–24.")

[18] Jemmott JB III, et al., Efficacy of a theory-based abstinence-only intervention over 24 months, Arch. Pediatr. Adolesc. Med. 164(2):152–9 (2010). Available online at

http://nationalabstinenceclearinghouse.com/pdf/contentmgmt/abstinence.pdf. (Jemmott et al. wrote: "The abstinence-only intervention compared with the health-promotion control intervention reduced by about 33% the percentage of students who ever reported having sexual intercourse by the time of the 24-month follow-up, controlling for grade, age, and intervention-maintenance condition.") Most studies report, however, that overall teen pregnancies are higher with abstinence-only education. See Stanger-Hall K. F. & Hall D. W., Abstinence-only education and teen pregnancy rates: Why we need comprehensive sex education in the U.S, PLoS One 6(10):e24658 (2011). Available online at https://www.ncbi.nlm.nih.gov/pmc/articles/PMC3194801/. (Stranger-Hall et al. wrote: "Using the most recent national data (2005) from all U.S. states with information on sex education laws or policies (N = 48), we show that increasing emphasis on abstinence education is positively correlated with teenage pregnancy and birth rates. This trend remains significant after accounting for socioeconomic status, teen educational attainment, ethnic composition of the teen population, and availability of Medicaid waivers for family planning services in each state. These data show clearly that abstinence-only education as a state policy is ineffective in preventing teenage pregnancy and may actually be contributing to the high teenage pregnancy rates in the U.S.")

[19] Data from CDC, Effectiveness of family planning methods [chart] (n.d.). Available online at https://www.cdc.gov/reproductivehealth/contraception/unintendedpregnancy/pdf/family-planning-methods-2014.pdf. Effectiveness as reported by CDC except as reported in next two notes.

[20] Although the CDC website reports a 22% failure rate for withdrawal, the latest research shows there has been a modest improvement to 20%. See Sundaram A., et al., Contraceptive failure in the United States: Estimates from the 2006–2010 National Survey of Family Growth, Perspec. Sex. Reprod. Health. 49(1):7–16 (2017). Available online at https://www.guttmacher.org/journals/psrh/2017/02/contraceptive-failure-united-states-estimates-2006-2010-national-survey-family.

[21] The CDC reports an 18% failure rate for the male condom, but Sundaram et al. (2017) (see endnote 20) reports some improvement to 13%. There has also been a small decline in failure rates for combined hormonal methods, but since these are not differentiated by type, we have not used those numbers.

[22] Trussell J., Contraceptive failure in the United States, Contraception 83(5):397–404 (2011). Available online at https://www.ncbi.nlm.nih.gov/pmc/articles/PMC3638209/. ("Not one of 15 clinical studies has reported an Implanon [an implantable contraceptive] failure. However, pregnancies during use of Implanon have been reported. We **arbitrarily** set the perfect-use and typical-use failure rates for Implanon at 0.05%" [reference citations omitted, emphasis added].) To obtain accurate failure rates of birth control methods of <1%, investigators must complete larger studies.

[23] BBC News, Implanon: 600 pregnancies despite contraceptive implant (2011). Available online at http://www.bbc.com/news/health-12117299. ("The implant maker, MSD, said no contraceptive was 100% effective. It added that unwanted pregnancies may occur if the implant was not correctly inserted, and said it had a failure rate of less than 1% if inserted correctly.")

[24] Abbasi J., Fertile gals look & sound more attractive: Study (2010). Available online at http://www.livescience.com/25457-fertile-women-attractiveness.html. (Abbasi wrote: "Men find women more attractive near ovulation, when they're most fertile, suggests the largest study yet to look at whether a gal's allure changes over the course of her menstrual cycle.")

[25] See RAINN, Victims of sexual violence: Statistics (https://www.rainn.org/statistics/victims-sexual-violence), reporting that one in six women is the victim of attempted or completed rape over her lifetime, and that one in ten rape victims is male. Female college students are three times more likely than women in general to experience sexual violence, and male college students are five times more likely than men in

general to experience sexual violence. Prison is also a very dangerous environment, as is the military. These numbers suggest that even if abstinence is your plan, a long-acting reversible birth control (LARC) method may still be a good backup plan.

[26] CDC, Reported cases of sexually transmitted diseases on the rise, some at alarming rate (2015). Available online at https://www.cdc.gov/nchhstp/newsroom/2015/std-surveillance-report-press-release.html. (The CDC reports: "Despite being a relatively small portion of the sexually active population, young people between the ages of 15 and 24 accounted for the highest rates of chlamydia and gonorrhea in 2014 and almost two thirds of all reported cases. Additionally, previous estimates suggest that young people in this age group acquire half of the estimated 20 million new STDs diagnosed each year.")

[27] Elbel F., U.S. birth rates and population growth (n.d.). Available online at http://www.susps.org/overview/birthrates.html. (Elbel wrote: "Each year there are approximately 4 million births in the U.S.")

[28] World Health Organization (WHO), Nonoxynol-9 ineffective in preventing HIV infection. Available online at http://www.who.int/mediacentre/news/notes/release55/en/. (Announcing findings by experts, WHO said that "two studies mentioned in the report point to an increased risk of sexually transmitted infections, including HIV infection, in women using nonoxynol-9 [spermicide] products. A possible reason, suggested by the findings of other studies, is that nonoxynol-9 can disrupt the epithelium, or wall, of the vagina, thereby potentially facilitating invasion by an infective organism. . . . The frequency of this epithelial disruption seems to depend on the intensity of use of the product—from 18% of women using the product every other day to 53% using it four times a day, in one study.")

[29] *Id.* (WHO reported: "Nonoxynol-9 is sometimes added to male condoms as a lubricant. The experts found no evidence that nonoxynol-9–lubricated condoms provided any more protection against pregnancy or sexually transmitted infections than condoms lubricated with silicone.")

[30] Modified from BruceBlaus and reprinted under a Creative Commons Attribution–Share Alike 4.0 International license at https://commons.wikimedia.org/wiki/File:Male_Condom.png.

[31] Modified from the Mayo Foundation at http://www.mayoclinic.org/tests-procedures/female-condom/multimedia/insertion-of-a-female-condom/img-20006788.

[32] Modified from Women's Health Advice at http://www.womens-health-advice.com/birth-control/diaphragm.html.

[33] Modified from FemCap at https://buyfemcap.com.

[34] See https://www.arhp.org/images/uploadDocs/nonchoosinggrg.pdf. (The Association of Reproductive Health Professionals wrote: "Effectiveness data for the first generation FemCap showed a failure rate of 14 percent among nulliparous women and 29 percent among women who have had a vaginal delivery.")

[35] Modified from the Mayo Clinic at http://www.mayoclinic.org/tests-procedures/contraceptive-sponge/details/what-you-can-expect/rec-20166803.

[36] Hayes T., 1.3 Million birth control pills recalled: Endo recalls 162 lots of subpotent birth control pills manufactured by Patheon, Healthcare Packaging (Nov. 14, 2016). Available online at https://www.healthcarepackaging.com/markets/pharmaceutical/news/13292260/13-million-birth-control-pills-recalled.

[37] PMS may be accompanied by moodiness, bloating, acne, breast tenderness, and fatigue.

[38] Modified from Captain Mums at https://www.captainmums.com/mums/birth-control-patch.

[39] Modified from the Mayo Clinic, available online at http://drugline.org/img/drug/nuvaring-ring-16801_1.jpg.

[40] Modified from www.livestrong.com. Credit: Mauricio Jordan de Souza Coelho/Hemera/Getty Images.

[41] Modified from the Mayo Clinic at http://www.mayoclinic.org/tests-procedures/contraceptive-implant/multimedia/insertion-of-implanon/img-20006795.

[42] Modified from Mayo Clinic, Mirena placement (1998–2020) at http://www.mayoclinic.org/tests-procedures/mirena/multimedia/mirena-placement/img-20006794.

[43] See Shapiro M., The IUD: What Do Gynecologists Know That Other Women Don't? LiveScience (2012), available online at http://www.livescience.com/21866-iud-gynecologists-birth-control-myths.html.

[44] Local School Health Advisory Council and Health Education Instruction. Tex. Educ. Code §28.004 (2019). https://statutes.capitol.texas.gov/Docs/ED/htm/ED.28.htm#28.004.

[45] Ducre K, Nine ways you can get an STD without having sex (2015). Available online at https://www.stdcheck.com/blog/how-to-get-an-std-without-having-sex/.

[46] Corlis N, How STDs can affect your baby and pregnancy (2015). Available online at https://www.stdcheck.com/blog/stds-that-can-affect-unborn-babies-pregnancy/.

[47] *Congenital* means having a trait, especially a disease or physical abnormality, since birth. Thus, *congenital syphilis* means having syphilis from birth.

[48] CDC, *Congenital syphilis—CDC Fact Sheet* (2017). Available online at https://www.cdc.gov/std/syphilis/stdfact-congenital-syphilis.htm.

[49] See CDC, *CDC fact sheet: Incidence, prevalence, and cost of sexually transmitted infections in the United States* (2013). Available online at https://www.cdc.gov/std/stats/sti-estimates-fact-sheet-feb-2013.pdf.

[50] Modified from FN 49.

[51] Wald A., Corey L., Persistence in the population: epidemiology, transmission. In: Arvin A., Campadelli-Fiume G., Mocarski E., et al., eds., *Human Herpesviruses: Biology, Therapy, and Immunoprophylaxis* (Cambridge: Cambridge University Press, 2007). Available online at https://www.ncbi.nlm.nih.gov/books/NBK47447/.

[52] *Id.*

[53] Modified from CDC, The low down on the most common STDs [A two-page chart]. Available online at https://www.gachd.org/gyt-get-yourself-tested/.

[54] See, for example, Corinna H., The buddy system: Effectiveness rates for backing up your birth control with a second method (1998–2020). Available online at http://www.scarleteen.com/article/sexual_health/the_buddy_system_effectiveness_rates_for_backing_up_your_birth_control_with_a_.

[55] Texas Freedom Network, Conspiracy of silence: Sexuality education in Texas public schools in 2015–2016. Available in 2017 online at https://tfn.org/new-tfn-education-fund-study-texas-is-failing-on-sex-education/, now available from Author.

[56] Teen Pregnancy Rate by State 2020, available online at https://worldpopulationreview.com/states/teen-pregnancy-rates-by-state/ ("Texas has the highest rate of repeat-teen births.")

[57] Power to Decide [formerly the National Campaign to Prevent Teen and Unplanned Pregnancy], Teen pregnancy rate comparison, 2013. Available online at https://powertodecide.org/what-we-do/information/national-state-data/teen-pregnancy-rate. The most recent data at Teen Pregnancy Rate by State 2020, available online at https://worldpopulationreview.com/states/teen-pregnancy-rates-by-state/ puts Texas at seventh place.

[58] See Henry J. Kaiser Family Foundation, The HIV/AIDS epidemic in the United States: The basics (2017). Available online at http://kff.org/hivaids/fact-sheet/the-hivaids-epidemic-in-the-united-states-the-basics/.

[59] Stanger-Hall K. F., & Hall, D. W., Abstinence-only education and teen pregnancy rates: Why we need comprehensive sex education in the U.S, PLoS One 6(10):e24658 (2011). Available online at https://www.ncbi.nlm.nih.gov/pmc/articles/PMC3194801/.

[60] Guttmacher Institute, American teens' sexual and reproductive health,(2016). Available online at https://www.sandersinstitute.com/blog/american-teens-sexual-and-reproductive-health-fact-sheet (Guttmacher wrote: "On average, young people in the United States have sex for the first time at about age 17 but do not marry until their mid-20s. During the interim period of nearly a decade or longer, they may be at heightened risk for unintended pregnancy and STIs. . . . The proportion of teens having sexual intercourse before age 15 has declined in recent years" [citations omitted].)

[61] Penman-Aguilar A., et al., Socioeconomic disadvantage as a social determinant of teen childbearing in the U.S., Public Health Rep. 128(Suppl 1):5–22 (2013). Available online at https://www.ncbi.nlm.nih.gov/pubmed/23450881. (Penman-Aguilar et al. wrote: "This review suggests that unfavorable socioeconomic conditions experienced at the community and family levels contribute to the high teen birth rate in the U.S.")

[62] See Boonstra H. D., What is behind the declines in teen pregnancy rates? Guttmacher Policy Review. 17(3) (2014). Available online at https://www.guttmacher.org/sites/default/files/pdfs/pubs/gpr/17/3/gpr170315.pdf. (Boonstra wrote:"Wide disparities in pregnancy rates by race and ethnicity persist, with rates among both black and Hispanic teens remaining twice as high as among their non-Hispanic white peers.")

[63] Strayhorn J. M., & Strayhorn J. C., Religiosity and teen birth rate in the United States, Reprod. Health. 17:6–14 (2009). Available online at https://reproductive-health-journal.biomedcentral.com/articles/10.1186/1742-4755-6-14. (Strayhorn and Strayhorn wrote: "With data aggregated at the state level, conservative religious beliefs strongly predict U.S. teen birth rates, in a relationship that does not appear to be the result of confounding by income or abortion rates. One possible explanation for this relationship is that teens in more religious communities may be less likely to use contraception.")

[64] See Boonstra H. D., What is behind the declines in teen pregnancy rates? Guttmacher Policy Review. 17(3) (2014). Available online at https://www.guttmacher.org/sites/default/files/pdfs/pubs/gpr/17/3/gpr170315.pdf. (Boonstra wrote: "After years of increases in the 1970s and 1980s, the teen pregnancy rate peaked in 1990 and has declined steadily since. Today, teen pregnancy, birth and abortion rates have reached historic lows. What is more, teen pregnancy rates have fallen in all 50 states and among all racial and ethnic groups.")

[65] *Id.* (Boonstra reported that "the decline in teen pregnancy since 2003 had little or nothing to do with teens' delaying sex. . . . Instead, the decline in teen pregnancy in recent years can be linked to improvements in teens' contraceptive use.")

www.ingramcontent.com/pod-product-compliance
Lightning Source LLC
Chambersburg PA
CBHW081311250726
48662CB00008B/2519